Advances in Cardiac and Pulmonary Rehabilitation

Advances in Cardiac and Pulmonary Rehabilitation

Mary C. Singleton and Eleanor F. Branch
Co-Editors

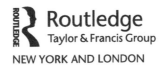

Routledge
Taylor & Francis Group
NEW YORK AND LONDON

First published 1990 by The Haworth Press, Inc.
10 Alice Street, Binghamton, NY 13904-1580

Published 2017 by Routledge
711 Third Avenue, New York, NY 10017, USA
2 Park Square, Milton Park, Abingdon, Oxfordshire OX14 4RN

First issued in paperback 2017

Routledge is an imprint of the Taylor & Francis Group, an informa business

Advances in Cardiac and Pulmonary Rehabilitation has also been published as *Physical Therapy in Health Care*, Volume 3, Numbers 1/2 1989.

Library of Congress Cataloging-in-Publication Data

Advances in cardiac and pulmonary rehabilitation / Mary C. Singleton and Eleanor F. Branch, co-editors.
    p. cm.
    "Has also been published as Physical therapy in health care, volume 3, numbers 1/2 1989" — T.p. verso.
    Based on papers originally presented at a conference sponsored by the Dept. of Physical Therapy of Duke University Medical Center, Durham, N.C., Apr. 15-16, 1988.
    Includes bibliographical references.
    ISBN 0-86656-986-3
    1. Lungs — Diseases — Physical therapy — Congresses. 2. Heart — Diseases — Physical therapy — Congresses. I. Singleton, Mary C. II. Branch, Eleanor F. III. Duke University. Dept. of Physical Therapy.
    [DNLM: 1. Heart Diseases — rehabilitation — congresses. 2. Lung diseases — rehabilitation — congresses. 3. Physical Therapy — congresses. W1]
RC735.P58A38   1989
616.2'406 — dc20
DNLM/DLC
for Library of Congress
89-24754
CIP

ISBN 13: 978-1-138-88144-0 (pbk)
ISBN 13: 978-0-86656-986-6 (hbk)

Advances in Cardiac and Pulmonary Rehabilitation

CONTENTS

ABOUT THE EDITORS

Mary C. Singleton, PhD, LPT, was formerly affiliated with the Department of Medical Allied Health Professions at the University of North Carolina at Chapel Hill. She is a member of the American Physical Therapy Association, the American Association for the Advancement of Science, and the American Association of Anatomists. She has published numerous articles in professional journals.

Eleanor F. Branch, PhD, LPT, is Associate Professor and Director of Graduate Studies in the Department of Physical Therapy at Duke University, Durham, North Carolina. She is a member of the American Physical Therapy Association. Dr. Branch has published articles in a number of professional journals.

Foreword

Physical therapists are assuming increasing responsibility in the organization and implementation of pulmonary and cardiac rehabilitation programs. Reflective of this expanding involvement, a course entitled "Advances in Cardiac and Pulmonary Rehabilitation" was sponsored by the Department of Physical Therapy of Duke University Medical Center, Durham, North Carolina, on April 15 and 16, 1988.

This collection is devoted to a series of essays derived from papers originally presented at that conference (with the exception of Ms. DeArmott's article). These essays mirror the ideas and experiences of individuals associated with a particular institution; however, the editors believe that the information presented can be of real value to health professionals in other settings—professionals, including physical therapists, who are, or who wish to become, involved in the care of patients with cardiac or chronic pulmonary disorders.

Pulmonary Rehabilitation:
Current Status and Future Trends

Neil R. MacIntyre, MD

SUMMARY. Pulmonary rehabilitation is a relatively new approach to the treatment of patients with chronic lung disease. These programs are designed to maximize the functional capabilities of such patients through a formal program of education, exercise, physical therapy, respiratory care and other modalities. Studies to date strongly suggest that pulmonary rehabilitation programs reduce morbidity (including medical costs) and improve the functional status of participants. However, programs are few in number and serve only a small fraction of the potential population. Moreover, reimbursement is often suboptimal. Research programs studying the cost effectiveness of various components of pulmonary rehabilitation urgently are needed to address these issues. From these will come guidelines and certification procedures that will allow more widespread development of truly effective programs; specifically, programs that will provide significant functional improvement at only a fraction of the resultant productivity increases and health care cost savings.

Pulmonary rehabilitation is a relatively new approach to the treatment of patients with chronic lung disease. Indeed, in the first half of this century, such patients usually were told to "take it easy," and they received minimal information on their disease process, on their medications, or on techniques to minimize symptoms and improve functional status. Patients thus were passive recipients of health care, and they did little to maximize what functional capabilities they may have had. More recently, comprehensive rehabilitation programs have changed dramatically this orientation to the long

---

Neil R. MacIntyre is Assistant Professor of Medicine at Duke University Medical Center, Box 3911, Durham, NC.

1

term care of patients with chronic lung disease.[1] The comments in this paper are an attempt to define where pulmonary rehabilitation is today, and where it can go over the next 20 years.

THE IMPACT OF CHRONIC LUNG DISEASE

It is estimated that about 10 million people in the United States have some form of chronic lung disease, most frequently chronic obstructive pulmonary disease (COPD), i.e., emphysema, chronic bronchitis and asthma.[2,3] There are, however, a smaller number of people with interstitial fibrosis, vascular diseases, and occupational diseases who also can be considered to have chronic lung disease.

Table 1 gives an idea of what chronic obstructive pulmonary disease costs the United States in terms of dollars.[4] Note from Table 1 that $3.3 billion a year is spent on direct health care. However, this is only a fraction of the actual cost to the U.S. economy. Specifically, since these people are disabled, they do not work or, if they do, they are not as productive as they should be. This lost productivity costs the economy an additional estimated $3.5 billion. Moreover, because there is a mortality associated with the disease, productivity is lost in that respect as well. Notice that the dollar loss to mortality is only about half what it is to morbidity (i.e., chronic lung disease does not kill people but rather disables them). Thus, although ten million people with chronic lung disease are fewer in number than those with cancer or heart disease, the prolonged mor-

TABLE 1. Chronic Lung Disease Costs (from Reference 4)

Chronic Obstructive Lung Disease

- Prevalence	10,000,000	
- Health care costs (direct)	$3.3 billion*	
- Lost earnings (morbidity)	$3.7 billion**	$8.8 billion
- Lost earnings (mortality)	$1.8 billion	

* Comparable to national costs for cancer

** Comparable to national losses for accidents

bidity of chronic lung disease makes the cost of it comparable to some of these more common diseases.

PULMONARY REHABILITATION: 1988

Statistics on the scope of pulmonary rehabilitation in 1988 are not readily available. Although Bickford and Hodgkin list 265 programs in the United States in 1987,[5] my own estimate would be that there are probably closer to 500 programs that offer some sort of pulmonary rehabilitation today. The Bickford and Hodgkin data also show that the average program serves 36 patients per year.[5] From this, we can thus estimate that approximately 18,000 people per year are enrolled in pulmonary rehabilitation programs. Note, however, that since there are about 10 million people with significant chronic lung disease, this figure means that we are exposing only a very small portion of the potential population to the benefits of pulmonary rehabilitation.

In terms of the program structure, Bickford and Hodgkin data demonstrate that there appear to be a number of different features offered.[5] Among the most common, however, is education. This component is felt to be very important in allowing the patient to "come to grips" with the disease, understand the disease, and thereby become more in control of the disease. Another common feature of pulmonary rehabilitation programs is exercise. This component is used both to improve ventilatory muscle function and to increase general cardiopulmonary fitness.[6] Other common components appear to be chest physical therapy, and respiratory care.

The average duration of pulmonary rehabilitation is reported to be 2 hrs/day, 2 to 2-1/2 days a week, for about 8 weeks.[5] Our own program at Duke runs 4 hours a day, 5 days a week and lasts 4-1/2 weeks. The average cost in the Bickford and Hodgkin survey was $1,200.[5] This ranged from a low of $35 (I presume one of these educational programs fell in that category) up to a high of $4,000 for a program that, I presume, has a fair amount of education and exercise in it.

In summary, Table 2 is an overview of what pulmonary rehabilitation looks like today. The important messages are that: (1) only a small fraction of the COPD population is being exposed to these

TABLE 2. Components of Pulmonary Rehabilitation (USA, 1987; from Reference 5)

```
Programs with:

      Pre-program spirometry       89%

      Pre-program exercise test     65%

      Education (lectures)          95%

      Exercise training             84%

      Smoking cessation             47%

      Physician team member         88%

Average duration      2.2 hours/day, 2.6 days/week, 8.3 weeks

Average cost          $1,232 ($35 - 4,000)
```

programs; and (2) what they are being exposed to consists of a lot of education, a fair amount of exercise, and a wide variety of program lengths and costs.

PULMONARY REHABILITATION — QUESTIONS FOR THE FUTURE

Two basic questions regarding the future of pulmonary rehabilitation come to mind: (1) Is pulmonary rehabilitation really cost effective? (2) If yes, how can the nation expand this service?

With regards to cost effectiveness, first we want to look at medical cost: Do we indeed reduce medical cost with a pulmonary rehabilitation programs? Second, do we improve productivity, reduce morbidity or change mortality with pulmonary rehabilitation programs? Data from large programs at Loma Linda and the University of Colorado are useful in assessing the effect on medical costs (see Figure 1).[7,8] Both of these studies report decreases in hospital days per year in patients after undergoing a pulmonary rehabilitation program. These studies, however, have been criticized for having a potential selection or recruitment bias towards an acutely ill population with a large number of inpatient hospital days (i.e., the natural history of chronic lung disease is over decades and thus baseline needs may not be reflected in the immediate recruitment period).

BENEFITS, LIMITATIONS, AND THE FUTURE OF PULMONARY REHABILITATION

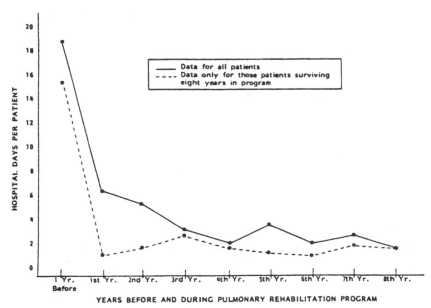

FIGURE 1. Analysis of hospital days before and during pulmonary rehabilitation program, Loma Linda University Medical Center. (reprinted with permission from Reference 6)

Nevertheless, the very substantial and persistent drop in hospital days would still suggest to me that pulmonary rehabilitation indeed makes a difference. Future studies, however, will have to assess carefully the long term pre-program medical costs and try to minimize, or at least account for, this potential selection bias.

What about productivity? Available data are limited although there is an interesting study from New York University in the early days of pulmonary rehabilitation programs that looked at functional status of patients 5 years after discharge from their program (see Table 3).[9] They reported results from 252 people with COPD who went through a pulmonary rehabilitation program. These were compared to 50 patients in their clinical records who had COPD. An obvious selection bias existed since the treated group consisted of patients motivated and interested and who were offered a rehabilita-

TABLE 3. Results of 5-Year Follow-up After Discharge (from Reference 9)

	Experimental Group (N = 252)	Control Group (N = 50)
Return to previous occupation, still working	6%	3%
Returned and placed in a job, still at work	13%	0%
Trained but never placed in a job	6%	0%
Able to care for self	19%	5%
Placed in a nursing home	8%	17%
Lost for unknown reasons	18%	27%
Died of respiratory failure	22%	42%
Died of unrelated causes	8%	6%

tion program, whereas the control population was obtained from historical records at a time when such programs were unavailable. Nevertheless, the pulmonary function tests in these two groups were rather similar and it is striking that the patients undergoing the rehabilitation program did have a higher proportion who were still working, a higher proportion who returned to work, a higher proportion who at least were trained for work, and a higher proportion that were able to care for themselves. Moreover, in the control group, a higher proportion ended up in nursing homes or died of respiratory failure.

Finally, a study from Denver looked at mortality in patients who went through a rehabilitation program and compared them with historical controls.[10] These data suggested that mortality is reduced by pulmonary rehabilitation programs. However, because of selection bias and the use of historical controls, this study is also open to criticism.

All of the above data, although tantalizing enough to keep us in the rehabilitation business, unfortunately are not so solid that programs have large referral patterns and are readily reimbursed by third party payers. So our first question then: "Is Pulmonary Rehabilitation Cost Effective?" cannot be clearly answered although I think all the evidence, faulted though it may be, clearly supports the concept that it is cost effective. Specifically, available data strongly suggest that pulmonary rehabilitation does reduce hospital days, does improve productivity and may reduce mortality.

If we believe that the data support the premise that pulmonary rehabilitation is cost effective, how do we expand this concept to a higher percentage of patients with chronic lung disease? To do this, I believe that a two-pronged approach is necessary. First, we have to generate better data. We really have to do proper studies to put these issues of cost effectiveness to rest. Second, we have to use these data to educate the health care system in order to construct certification procedures with health agencies, government agencies, and reimbursement groups.

As far as research needs, I think most importantly we need better long term follow up studies that carefully look at functional levels and productivity as well as health care costs. Unfortunately, I think they will need to be "pre vs. post" studies because randomized control studies are going to be impractical. Specifically, I don't think any of us would ever want to have a patient whom we believe could benefit from pulmonary rehabilitation flip a coin and have to be told, "I'm sorry, you will be in the control group and we'll just follow you for 10 years to see how badly you will do." Thus good randomized control studies just are not going to happen.

There are other important research needs as well. Specifically, I think we need data helping us to understand what are the effective components of pulmonary rehabilitation and what components merely add excess cost. Taking exercise as an example, it would be useful to document how important it is, if it is, to those 16 percent of programs that don't routinely include exercise programs (see Table 2). Moreover, clarification is needed as to what types of exercise and what magnitude of exercise are useful. Similar studies also need to be done on other common components of pulmonary rehabilitation programs, such as physical therapy and respiratory care. We also don't know the optimal role of nutrition in a pulmonary rehabilitation program. Specifically, how important are metabolic measurements and dietary manipulations of fats, carbohydrates, and proteins? From a psychosocial point of view, we need to ask: what is the role of psychological assessment and treatment in chronic lung disease? What is the importance of occupational therapy?

Research on newer or less common rehabilitation components also needs to be done. For instance, should transtracheal O_2 insertion be incorporated into rehabilitation programs? Should intermittent mechanical ventilation be included? With regard to this latter modality, the concept exists that people with chronically fatigued diaphragms might benefit from diaphragm rest at night with mechanical ventilation. Much more research is needed into respiratory muscle function in chronic disease to answer this question.

Finally, I think research needs to look at predictors of success. Clearly there are some patients who, regardless of their treatment program, will not do well. Conversely, there are others who appear debilitated and "end stage" at the beginning of a program but who can do extremely well. I have been struck in my own program that pulmonary function tests are not always very good predictors of performance in a pulmonary rehabilitation program. Some of our best results have had some of the worst spirometric values and, conversely, some of our poorest results have actually had very good spirometric values. Indeed, psychology and psychological tests scores as an index of motivation may offer a far more important set of predictors. From these should come very important selection criteria for future programs. The net result of all of these studies should allow us to construct optimal cost effective programs for the patients we serve.

The second "prong" in the attack of advancing pulmonary rehabilitation is certification. Once the data are solid, and effective components of pulmonary rehabilitation are clear, the logical next step is to become certified by the scientific community, government and third party payer groups. This will help tremendously in public recognition, in physician referral, in providing guidelines for the development of new programs, and, finally, in reimbursement. Voluntary health organizations might be a useful place to start (perhaps modelled after American Thoracic Society blood gas and pulmonary function standards). From there, governmental certification would seem desirable. At the present time, some states have certification procedures for cardiac rehabilitation. In my own state of North Carolina, this is being expanded to cardiopulmonary rehabilitation certification. I think that will be a very big step forward with the reimbursing communities. Medicare already recognizes outpatient pulmonary rehabilitation in certified comprehensive outpatient rehabilitation facilities (CORFs).[11] These include respiratory care, physical therapy, and exercise for chronic lung disease. The bottom line in reimbursement, however, is each insurer. Unfortunately, since there are several thousand such companies in this country, there are several thousand different rules and regulations regarding pulmonary rehabilitation. Again, I think certification will help with this insurance reimbursement problem.

PULMONARY REHABILITATION — THE FUTURE

So where is pulmonary rehabilitation going over the next 20 years? If proper research confirms its apparent cost effectiveness, then certification and reimbursement will follow. Under these circumstances, the current 500 programs could expand several-fold and begin to equal in number the more established cardiac and neuromuscular rehabilitation programs in the United States. Patient enrollment should increase accordingly and we might then begin to make a significant impact on the detrimental long term consequences of chronic lung disease. All of this should be accomplished at program costs that are a fraction of resultant productivity and health care cost savings.

REFERENCES

1. ATS Position Statement on Pulmonary Rehabilitation. *Am. Rev. Resp. Dis.* 124:663, 1981.

2. Prevalence of selected chronic respiratory conditions — 1970. NCHS Vital and Health Statistics, Series 10, No. 84. DHEW Publication No. (HRA) 74-1511, 1973.

3. Respiratory disease task force report on prevention, control and education. DHEW Publication No. NIH 77-1248, 1977.

4. Luce, BR et al. Smoking and alcohol abuse: A comparison of their economic consequences. *N. Engl. J. Med.* 298:569-571, 1978.

5. Bickford, LS, Hodgkin JE. National pulmonary rehabilitation survey. *Respiratory Care* 33:1030-1035, 1988.

6. Holle, RHO et al. Increased Muscle Efficiency and Sustained Benefits in an Outpatient Community Hospital-Based Pulmonary Rehabilitation Program. *Chest* 94:1161-1168, 1988.

7. Hodgkin, JE, Branscomb BV, Anholm, JD, Gray LS. Benefits limitations and the future of pulmonary rehabilitation. Chapter 24 in Hodgkin, JE, Zorn EG, Connors GL (eds) *Pulmonary rehabilitation—guideline to success.* Butterworth Publishers, Boston, 1984.

8. Hudson LD et al. Hospitalization needs during an outpatient rehabilitation program for severe chronic airway obstruction. *Chest* 70:606-610, 1976.

9. Haas, A et al. Rehabilitation in chronic obstructive pulmonary disease: A 5 year study of 252 male patients. *Med Clinics of North America* 53:593-606, 1969.

10. Pulmonary Rehabilitation Study Group, TL Petty chairman. Community resources for rehabilitation of patients with chronic obstructive pulmonary disease and cor pulmonale. *Circ.* 49 (supplement A1-20), 1974.

11. Medicare Program; Comprehensive Outpatient Rehabilitation Facility Services (Sec. 933, PL96-499). Federal Register, May 10, 1982.

Pulmonary Rehabilitation: Mechanisms of Benefits

Nelson E. Leatherman, PhD
Neil R. MacIntyre, MD

SUMMARY. Pulmonary rehabilitation increases exercise tolerance and improves general well-being of patients with chronic lung disease. The mechanisms of these benefits, however, are not clear. This paper will review the rationale and supporting data for physiologic and psychologic mechanisms that may be operative in the pulmonary rehabilitation process. Pre and post physiologic and psychologic test data obtained from 79 participants in the Duke intensive pulmonary rehabilitation program are presented and serve to demonstrate the benefits of pulmonary rehabilitation. Hypothetical physiologic responses to progressive exercise are considered for four potential mechanisms; exercise training, increased motivation, decreased hyperventilation, and improved efficiency. The pattern of changes in test data suggests that the benefits derived from our rehabilitation program occur primarily as a result of exercise training, and, to a lesser extent, from increased efficiency and better airway management.

GOAL OF PULMONARY REHABILITATION

As stated by the American Thoracic Society (ATS), the goal of pulmonary rehabilitation is to "return the patient to the highest possible functional capacity allowed by his pulmonary handicap and overall life situation."[1] Pulmonary rehabilitation thus is not designed to cure the lung disease; rather, it is designed to treat the

---

Nelson E. Leatherman is Medical Research Associate and Director, Pulmonary Rehabilitation, Box 3861, Duke University Medical Center, Durham, NC 27710. Neil R. MacIntyre is Assistant Professor of Medicine, Box 3911, Duke University Medical Center.

11

ventilation and gas exchange abnormalities that exist and maximize the functional capacity. That pulmonary rehabilitation can attain this goal seems clear. What is not clear, however, are the mechanisms by which this takes place. The purpose of this paper is to review both the rationale and supporting data for various physiologic and psychologic mechanisms that may be operative in the rehabilitation process.

MECHANISMS OF FUNCTIONAL DETERIORATION IN CHRONIC LUNG DISEASE

Chronic lung disease progressively damages lung tissue and airways and, over a period of years, ultimately results in a depletion of ventilatory reserves. Complicating this physiologically are abnormalities in gas exchange and elevations in pulmonary vascular pressures that lead to right ventricular dysfunction. All of these factors contribute to the sensation of dyspnea and the resultant limitation on physical activity.

As dyspnea and exercise capacity worsen, the need for medical care increases and a confusing combination of functional limitations and dependence on others is thrust upon the patient. The net effect is a profound sense of "loss of control" with consequent depression and anxiety.

All of these factors are further worsened by what I will refer to as the vicious cycle of inactivity (Figure 1). The cycle begins when the patient starts to associate exertional dyspnea with the disease and no longer recognizes dyspnea as a normal response to exertion. In this setting, exertional dyspnea promotes increased levels of anxiety, depression, and fear of exertion, all of which generally lead to physical inactivity. The lack of exercise, in turn, leads to both central and peripheral deconditioning and, ultimately, to decreased endurance, weakness, and often to muscular atrophy. As a result of deconditioning, the patient develops greater dyspnea, an even greater intolerance to exertion, and further loss of functional capacity. As the cycle continues, the patient's exercise capacity spirals progressively downward while the levels of fear, anxiety and depression increase unabated, and the patient becomes progressively psychologically and physically incapacitated. This progressive loss

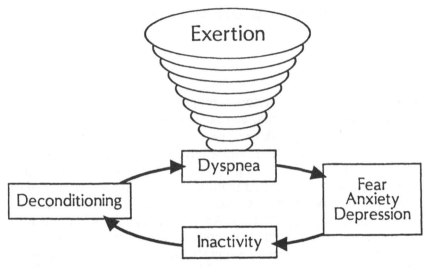

FIGURE 1. Vicious cycle of inactivity.

of exercise capacity resulting from the vicious cycle of inactivity is superimposed on the underlying functional reduction caused by the lung disease. While the limitation to exercise imposed by the lung disease is generally considered irreversible, the additional functional deterioration caused by physiologic and psychologic changes associated with the cycle of inactivity are considered reversible.

OBJECTIVE MANIFESTATIONS OF FUNCTIONAL DETERIORATION IN CHRONIC LUNG DISEASE

Exercise Tests

Testing exercise capacity is one of the best objective ways to measure functional physical capabilities. The physiologic response to exercise usually is obtained by performing progressive exercise on a treadmill or stationary bicycle. The exercise is performed to exhaustion or to a symptom limitation while oxygen uptake (VO_2), heart rate (HR), and ventilation (VE) are measured. Before reviewing the abnormal response of chronic lung disease patients to such exercise, it would be useful to review the response in healthy individuals.

Healthy Subjects

When an individual performs progressive exercise, the VO_2 increases until the individual can no longer perform the work load. The increase in VO_2 with exercise is due to increases in heart rate (HR), stroke volume (SV), and arterial-venous oxygen difference ($VO_2 = HR^*SV^* (A - V)O_2$). The healthy, motivated subject stops exercise because of an inability to maintain aerobic metabolism; VO_2 is maximal in this situation (Figure 2a) and is referred to as the aerobic capacity (VO_{2max}). An aerobic capacity within the normal predicted range implies a normal exercise capacity, while reduction in aerobic capacity suggests an exercise limiting impairment. The VO_2 response thus provides information as to whether or not the exercise capacity is impaired. If impaired, the factors limiting the exercise (i.e., reduced cardiac or ventilatory reserves) must then be determined from the HR and VE responses.

The heart rate response (Figure 2b) provides a means of assessing the cardiac reserve during progressive exercise. Since the stroke volume is maximized at relatively low work rates, the increase in cardiac output necessary to meet the demands of progressive exercise depends primarily on increases in heart rate. When HR increases to a physiological maximum (i.e., predicted maximal heart rate), cardiac output is also maximal. At HR_{max}, there is no cardiac reserve to support the increasing work load (cardiovascular limitation). Depletion of cardiac reserves, therefore, is signaled by the exercise heart rate increasing to the predicted maximal HR, as shown in Figure 2b.

The ventilatory response (Figure 2c) provides a means of assessing ventilatory reserve. Exercise ventilation (VE) increases with work rate, slowly at first but more rapidly toward the end of the exercise. The acceleration in ventilation in the later phases of exhausting exercise is caused by the additional CO_2 load resulting from buffering of excess lactic acid produced by anaerobic metabolism (AT = anaerobic threshold, Figure 2c). The magnitude of the ventilatory reserve is determined by comparing the peak exercise

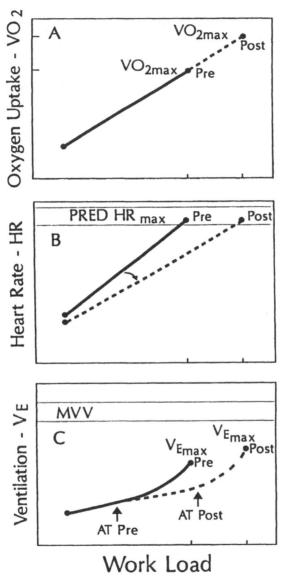

FIGURE 2. Physiologic response to progressive exercise in healthy subjects. Panels A, B, and C show oxygen uptake (VO_2), heart rate (HR), and minute ventilation (VE) respectively versus work load. The solid line (——) represents the response prior to physical training. The dotted line (---) represents the response after physical training.

ventilation to the maximum voluntary ventilation (MVV) obtained during pulmonary function testing. As shown in Figure 2c, VE_{max} is usually only 50% to 80% of the MVV in the healthy, motivated individual at the end of exhausting exercise, implying that the ventilatory reserves are not depleted and that there is no ventilatory limitation to exercise.

In summary, healthy subjects have a normal aerobic capacity, but have a cardiovascular limitation to exercise. While they may experience exertional dyspnea, at exhaustion they still have significant ventilatory reserve. These responses are in marked distinction to those observed in patients with chronic pulmonary disease.

Pulmonary Patients

When the pulmonary patient performs progressive exercise, oxygen uptake increases until the patient can no longer perform the work load. Unlike the healthy, motivated individual who stops exercising because of depletion of cardiac reserves and exhaustion, pulmonary patients usually stop the progressive exercise as a result of symptom limitations. Such limitations may occur because of severe shortness of breath, fear of exertion, or a lack of motivation. The peak VO_2 in symptom limited patients is less than maximal (Figure 3a) and is referred to as the symptom-limited oxygen consumption (VO_{2SL}) to differentiate it from the aerobic capacity (VO_{2max}); the latter is not possible to accurately determine in such patients because of the onset of symptoms.

Heart rate increases with work load (Figure 3b), but, unlike that in the healthy individual, usually does not reach the predicted maximum. In this situation, the cardiac reserve is not depleted and, therefore, there is no cardiovascular limitation to exercise. Occasionally the pulmonary patient's symptom limited heart rate (HR_{SL}) does reach the predicted maximum HR. Then, as with the healthy individual, cardiac output is maximal, cardiac reserves are depleted, and a cardiovascular limit is reached. In the setting of significant pulmonary disease, this may reflect right ventricular dysfunction.

Figure 3c, unlabeled solid line, shows that, in pulmonary patients, ventilation increases with work load and usually reaches a

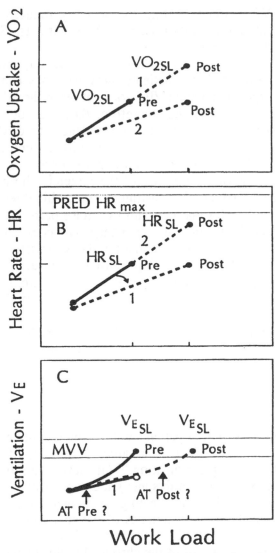

FIGURE 3. Physiologic respone to progressive exercise in pulmonary patients. Panels A, B, and C show oxygen uptake (VO₂), heart rate (HR), and minute ventilation (VE) respectively versus work load. The solid line (⎯⎯) represents a respone prior to rehabilitation, while the dotted line (---) represents a response after rehabilitation. The paths labelled 1 or 2 depend on the mechanism involved in producing the increase in work load after rehabilitation and are described in detail in the text.

maximum (VE_{SL}) approximating the severely reduced maximum voluntary ventilation (MVV) seen in these patients. Since additional ventilation is not available to support the demands of the progressive exercise, ventilatory reserve is depleted, and a ventilatory limit is reached. Some patients, however, may demonstrate a ventilatory response in which VE_{SL} does not reach the MVV (Figure 3c, path 1, open circle) and, therefore, they are not ventilatory-limited. If these latter patients show no evidence of a cardiovascular or gas exchange limitation, the factors most likely limiting exercise are either fear of exertion, lack of motivation, or hypersensitivity to dyspnea. Because of the severity of their exercise limitation, pulmonary patients may not demonstrate an anaerobic threshold (AT).

An additional factor that may limit exercise performance in pulmonary patients is impaired gas exchange. A gas exchange limitation presents itself as a reduction in arterial oxygen saturation below a level of 88% ($P_aO_2 < 55$ mm Hg) during exercise.

In summary, the physiologic response for the pulmonary patient may show an impaired oxygen uptake because of a ventilatory limitation, a cardiovascular limitation, a gas exchange limitation, or a nonspecific limitation such as a lack of motivation, fear of exertion, or hypersensitivity to dyspnea. Each of these limitations may occur singly or in combination.

Psychologic Tests

Psychological testing of patients with chronic pulmonary disease inevitably demonstrates depression, anxiety, fatigue, difficulty with coping, and somatic preoccupation.[6,7] Of these, the most common findings are anxiety (fear of dyspnea) and depression characterized by pessimism of outlook and feelings of hopelessness and worthlessness. While these characteristics of patients with chronic lung disease differ dramatically from the norm, little differentiation can be made from other groups of the chronically physically ill.[8] Those psychological tests emphasizing "loss of control" over life, "dependence" on others, and "inability to cope" always are markedly abnormal in patients with chronic pulmonary disease. Psychological admissions in COPD patients are always higher and suicide rates are seven-fold that of a control population.

EVIDENCE THAT PULMONARY REHABILITATION PROGRAMS REVERSE FUNCTIONAL DETERIORATION

Some of the most recent data supporting the concept that pulmonary rehabilitation reverses functional deterioration come from our own program at Duke University Medical Center. The psychological and physiological data to be presented here were obtained from 79 pulmonary patients participating in the intensive out-patient Pulmonary Rehabilitation Program. The program is a 4 1/2 week intensive, multi-disciplinary program that meets 4 hours per day, 5 days per week. The program, the goal of which is consistent with the ATS statement on pulmonary rehabilitation, provides bronchial hygiene, medication optimization, education, exercise, and psychological support. The daily exercise routine consists of 1 1/2 to 2 hours (excluding rest periods) of a combination of floor exercises, arm and leg ergometry, walking, Nautilus exercise, inspiratory muscle training, and pool exercises. Psychological assessment and consultation is provided by a staff psychologist through both individual and group sessions.

Psychologic Changes

Psychological changes resulting from the Duke pulmonary rehabilitation program are assessed by the Psychological General Well-Being Index (PGWB) designed by Dupuy.[2] The PGWB is a 22 item, self-report questionnaire tapping 6 dimensions of psychological functioning including anxiety, depressed mood, positive well-being, self-control, general health, and vitality. Individual items are scored from 0 to 5 with higher scores indicating greater well-being. In addition, a summary score having a maximum of 110 is derived by summing the individual item scores.

Figure 4 shows the changes in the mean PGWB index and the means of the six subscales of the 79 patients expressed as a percent of the normal score, as the result of completion of the rehabilitation program. The average raw PGWB index was 60 (73%) upon entry into the Duke program and 78 (95%) on discharge compared to to 82 (100%) in the normal population; a 30% improvement in the psychological index. Scores on all six subscales increased after rehabilitation, with many approaching the norm by the end of the

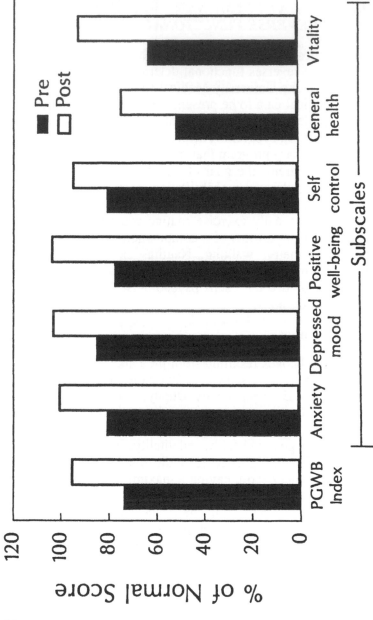

FIGURE 4. Results of administering the Psychological General Well-Being (PGWB) schedule before (closed bars) and after (open bars) intensive pulmonary rehabilitation.

20

program. Major contributions to the total index came from the subscales of vitality, positive well-being, anxiety and general health. The general health subscale, while showing significant improvement, remained notably below normal suggesting that, as a whole, the patients retain a view of their state of health which is consistent with their condition. They have a chronic lung disease, they recognize that fact, and yet they are able to deal better with their chronic disease after the rehabilitation process.

The documented changes in the PGWB index and its subscales suggest that the patients' improved sense of well-being and self-esteem may be related to positive changes in their psychological state. It is plausible that these same changes in the psychologic state may also account for the improved exercise capacity by improving motivation, reducing fear of exertion, and desensitizing the patient to shortness of breath.

Physiologic Changes

Figure 5 shows a preliminary compilation of data illustrating the effects of pulmonary rehabilitation on a variety of physiologic measurements. There was a 44% increase in the distance covered during the 12 minute walk test, and a 20% improvement in the work load obtained during a progressive cardiopulmonary stress test; this reflected a statistically significant increase in exercise capacity. The improvement in work load represents a 41% increase in the total work performed.

Data derived from the pulmonary function tests; (i.e., the forced expired volume in 1 second [FEV1.0], forced vital capacity [FVC], and maximum voluntary ventilation [MVV]) showed that there was no significant change in either the FVC or the FEV1.0 as a result of pulmonary rehabilitation. Although the maximum voluntary ventilation (MVV) increased about 9%, this increase also was not statistically significant. It should be noted that some individuals did experience improvement in pulmonary function; this improvement was considered the direct result of optimizing the individual's pulmonary medications during the course of the program.

As a result of the rehabilitation program, VO_{2SL} increased 15% and VE_{SL} increased 13%; however, there was no significant change

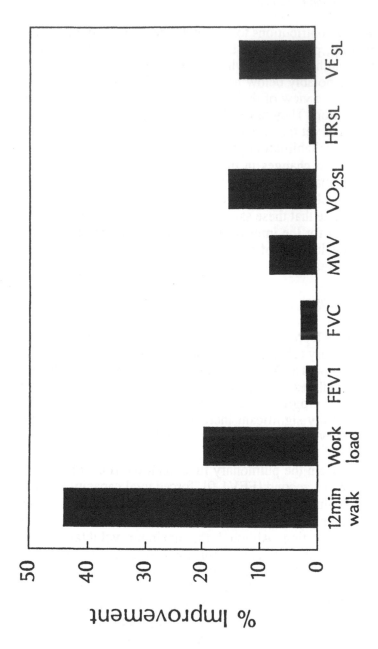

FIGURE 5. Percent change in various measures of exercise capacity and pulmonary function after intensive pulmonary rehabilitation.

in HR$_{SL}$ after completion of the program. Our findings of a significant increase in oxygen uptake without a significant change in maximum heart rate strongly suggest that the patients are indeed experiencing a physical training effect. Such a training effect may be one of the mechanisms by which pulmonary rehabilitation helps to reverse functional deterioration of pulmonary patients.

MECHANISMS WHEREBY PULMONARY REHABILITATION ACCOMPLISHES THE REVERSAL IN FUNCTIONAL DETERIORATION

How might the documented psychologic and physiologic changes just described for patients in our program be explained? The remainder of this paper will consider some of the real and hypothetical mechanisms that may be at work here.

In 1973, Agle et al.[3] summarized mechanisms that they felt were central to the improvement in psychologic state and performance of COPD patients. More recently, Belman[4] suggested five such mechanisms to account for the observed improvement in exercise tolerance: (1) improved aerobic capacity, (2) increased motivation, (3) desensitization to the sensation of dyspnea, (4) improved ventilatory muscle function and (5) improved techniques of performance. While numerous studies have provided evidence supporting one or more of these factors, none has yet emerged as the predominant mechanism. Indeed, these mechanisms probably operate in combination depending on both the individual and the specific strengths of the rehabilitation program. In this discussion, we will consider specifically the hypothetical role of exercise training, increased motivation, decreased hyperventilation, and increased efficiency in the production of the psychologic and physiologic changes seen in our patients undergoing pulmonary rehabilitation.

Exercise Training

Prior to discussing exercise training in pulmonary patients, it is informative to consider the physiologic changes resulting from physical training in healthy subjects. After physical training, the healthy subject has a greater maximal oxygen uptake (aerobic capacity), as shown by the dotted line in Figure 2a, and thus he can exercise to a higher work load. The increase in VO_{2max} is the result of an increased maximum cardiac output (O_2 transport) and a greater arterial-venous oxygen difference (O_2 extraction). The maximum cardiac output increases solely as a result of an increase in the stroke volume since the maximum heart rate does not change significantly with physical training, as shown in Figure 2b, dotted line. The slope of the HR response, however, decreases so that at any submaximal work load, a lower heart rate (and, presumably, a lower cardiac output) is required after training. The combination of an increase in VO_{2max} without a change in HR_{max} causes the O_2 pulse to increase (O_2 pulse $= VO_{2max}/HR_{max}$). The ventilatory response (Figure 2c, dotted line) shows that after physical training the anaerobic threshold (AT) occurs at a higher work load both in absolute terms and as a percent of the maximum work that can be attained. Although VE_{max} may increase after training, there is still ventilatory reserve. These physiological changes are typical of the training response in healthy individuals.

The existence of a training effect in pulmonary patients is a controversial issue. Since it is generally considered necessary to exercise at an intensity approximating the anaerobic threshold in order to experience a training effect, moderate to severely impaired pulmonary patients reportedly are unable to experience either cardiovascular or muscular conditioning because they may become symptom-limited prior to developing a significant lactic acidosis.[5] Less severely impaired patients, however, do develop a significant lactic acidosis during progressive exercise, and still others may develop localized metabolic acidosis that is sufficient to promote the training effect.

If exercise training is a primary mechanism by which the patient's functional capacity increases after rehabilitation, the pattern of the physiologic response would be similar to that observed in healthy subjects. The VO_{2SL} would increase as shown in Figure 3a, path 1. The slope of the heart rate response would decrease with training as shown in Figure 3b, path 1 and there would be no significant change in HR_{SL}. If HR_{SL} were to increase during rehabilitation, the improved work capacity could still be ascribed to a training effect only if VO_{2SL} increased in excess of any increase in HR_{SL}. In pulmonary patients then, as in healthy subjects, an increase in O_2 pulse (VO_{2SL}/HR_{SL}) is evidence of a training effect. Figure 3c, dotted line, shows that an increase in the anaerobic threshold (AT) as a result of training would allow the patient to continue breathing at a higher work load in spite of the fixed ventilatory limit.

Increased Motivation

Lack of motivation is a factor that similarly may reduce exercise tolerance and limit exercise. Characteristically, this factor is important whenever the physiologic response demonstrates neither a cardiovascular, ventilatory, nor gas exchange limitation to exercise. Under these conditions, neither cardiac nor ventilatory reserves would be depleted (Figure 3b, solid line, and Figure 3c, path 1, solid line). Increased motivation after the rehabilitation intervention would allow the patient to utilize these reserves. HR_{SL} would increase toward the predicted HR_{max} as shown in Figure 3b, path 2, and VE_{SL} would increase from the open circle toward the MVV without a change in the AT (Figure 3c, dotted line). The O_2 pulse would not change significantly with this mechanism because VO_{2SL} would increase in proportion to HR_{SL} as shown in Figure 3a, path 1.

Decreased Hyperventilation

Anxiety in the pulmonary patient is often expressed as pronounced fear of exertion or shortness of breath and may be evidenced by hyperventilation during any form of exertion. During progressive exercise the MVV would be reached earlier because of this hyperventilation, thereby limiting the maximum work load attained. This situation, which is represented by the unlabeled solid line in Figure 3c, can be identified by the development of a respiratory alkalosis during exercise. After rehabilitation, reduction in anxiety would allow ventilation to increase more in accord with metabolic demand (Figure 3c, dotted line). Ventilation would be reduced at any given work rate thereby reducing the respiratory alkalosis and VE_{SL} would increase toward the limiting MVV. The symptom limited heart rate (HR_{SL}) would increase along path 2, Figure 3b, to provide the increment in maximum cardiac output necessary for the increase in VO_{2SL} shown in Figure 3a, path 1, and, consequently, there would be no change in O_2 pulse.

Increased Efficiency

Another mechanism that might be associated with pulmonary rehabilitation is increased efficiency. This mechanism would allow the individual's exercise capacity to improve without a corresponding increase in VO_{2SL} (Figure 3a, path 2). At any given work load, the patient would be able to exercise with a lower oxygen consumption than prior to rehabilitation. Since the energy requirements (VO_{2SL}) and, consequently, maximum cardiac output, would remain unchanged, no significant change would be expected in HR_{SL} (Figure 3b, path 1) or the O_2 pulse. Although the ventilatory response (Figure 3c, dotted line) would also be more efficient (lower ventilation required for a given submaximum work rate) after rehabilitation, the AT would not increase with improved efficiency, and VE_{SL} would be unable to change because of the fixed ventilatory limit. This physiologic response typifies improved efficiency and has been reported as a mechanism by which exercise tolerance is improved in pulmonary patients.[3,5]

In addition to the increase in exercise tolerance resulting from the four mechanisms described above, several other factors probably contribute to the patient's increased feeling of well-being. Among these are a better understanding of his disease process, a firmer grasp on the role of medications and how to adjust them, and a realistic outlook for the future. All of these factors tend to return control to the patient, lessen dependence, and improve his ability to cope.

SUMMARY OF MECHANISMS RELATED TO FUNCTIONAL IMPROVEMENT DURING PULMONARY REHABILITATION

Table 1 summarizes the pattern of hypothetical physiologic changes that characterize each of the four mechanisms discussed. With this in mind, it becomes possible to identify the mechanisms responsible for the increased exercise tolerance in the Duke partici-

TABLE 1. Hypothetical changes in physiologic response due to rehabilitation. Characteristic changes in VO_{2SL}, HR_{SL}, O_2 pulse, and VE_{SL} are indicated for each of the four mechanisms discussed. Increases are represented by ($\uparrow$) while no change is represented by ($\ominus$).

	Training Effect	Increased Motivation	Decreased Hyperventilation	Increased Efficiency
$VO_{2\ SL}$	$\uparrow$	$\uparrow$	$\uparrow$	$\ominus$
HR_{SL}	$\ominus$	$\uparrow$	$\uparrow$	$\ominus$
$O_{2\ pulse}$	$\uparrow$	$\ominus$	$\ominus$	$\ominus$
$V_{E\ SL}$	$\ominus$	$\uparrow$	$\ominus$	$\ominus$

pants. The increase in O_2 pulse resulting from the 15% increase in VO_{2SL} and the insignificant change in HR_{SL} (Figure 5) strongly suggest that the primary mechanism responsible for the increased work capacity observed in the Duke program is a training effect. As shown on Table 1, increased O_2 pulse is not characteristic of the other three mechanisms. The disproportionate increase in work load (20%) over VO_{2SL} (15%) seen in our patients (Figure 5), however, does suggest a small contribution to the improved exercise tolerance may have resulted from improved efficiency as improved efficiency is the only other mechanism that characteristically shows no increase in HR_{SL}. The 13% increase in VE_{SL} (Figure 5) is consistent with the other physiologic data only if the ventilatory reserve increased during rehabilitation. Although the 9% increase in MVV thought to be the result of better airway management was not statistically significant, it provides the increase in ventilatory reserve necessary to explain most of the increase in VE_{SL}.

The improved exercise capacity observed in our group of patients appears to have been primarily the result of an improved physical condition and, to a lesser extent, improved efficiency and better airway management.

This analysis demonstrates the usefulness of the physiologic exercise response in identifying the beneficial mechanisms in pulmo- nary rehabilitation. Even greater use may be found in systematically identifying individual patient's limitations to exercise, then individ- ualizing the rehabilitation program so as to best use the appropriate physiologic and psychologic mechanisms to reduce those limita- tions.

CONCLUSIONS

Both rationale and evidence exist for considering physiologic and psychologic mechanisms for the functional benefits derived from pulmonary rehabilitation. The rationale lies in the sequence of physiological and psychological changes that constitute the vicious cycle of inactivity and consideration of how to best reverse that cycle. Evidence abounds in the form of both psychologic and physi- ologic data obtained before and after a rehabilitation intervention. Having now identified numerous plausible mechanisms, we must develop our skills in analyzing and interpreting the data to better define the patient's limitations and, then decide how to individual- ize the pulmonary rehabilitation program to facilitate the appropri- ate mechanisms.

REFERENCES

1. Pulmonary Rehabilitation: Official American Thoracic Society Statement. Am. Rev. Respir. Dis., 124:663-666, 1981

2. Dupuy, H.J.: The Psychological General Well-Being (PGWB) Index. In: Wenger, Nanette et al. (eds.): Assessment of Quality of Life in Clinical Trials of Cardiovascular Therapies. LeJacq Publishing Inc., 1984, p.170-183

3. Agle, D.P., Baum, G.L., Chester, I.H. et al.: Multi-discipline Treatment of Chronic Pulmonary Insufficiency: Functional Status at One Year Follow-up. In: Johnston, R.F. (ed.): Pulmonary Medicine: A Hahnemann Symposium. New York, Grune and Stratton, 1973, p.355

4. Belman, M.J.: Exercise in Chronic Obstructive Pulmonary Disease. Clinics in Chest Medicine, 7(4):585-597, 1986

5. Hodgkin, J.E. (ed.): Chronic Pulmonary Disease: Current Concepts in Di- agnosis and Comprehensive Care. Park Ridge, Illinois, American College of Chest Physicians, 1979

6. Agle, D.P., and Baum, G.L.: Psychological Aspects of Chronic Obstruc- tive Pulmonary Disease. Med. Clin. North Am., 61:749-758, 1977

7. Dudley, D.L., Glaser, E.M., Jorgenson, B. et al.: Psychosocial Concomitants to Rehabilitation in Chronic Obstructive Pulmonary Disease. Part I. Psychosocial and Psychological Considerations. Chest, 77:413-420, 1980

8. De Cencio, D.V., Leshner, M., Leshner, B. et al.: Personality Characteristics of Patients with Chronic Obstructive Pulmonary Emphysema. Arch. Phys. Med. Rehab., 49:471-475, 1968

Pulmonary Rehabilitation During Acute Hospitalization

Theresa G. Davidson, MS, PT

SUMMARY. Patients with chronic obstructive pulmonary disease cannot reverse their disease process but can do much to improve functional abilities through pulmonary rehabilitation. A program that is conducted in the acute care setting at Duke University Medical Center is described in this paper. It consists of education, breathing retraining, exercise, and initiation of an aerobic-style walking or bicycling program. The use of supplemental oxygen and oximetry also are discussed.

INTRODUCTION

Pulmonary rehabilitation has been defined by the American Thoracic Society as a comprehensive program aimed at improving the functioning ability of the patient with chronic pulmonary disease.[1] To attempt to achieve this with an individual hospitalized because of an acute exacerbation of his baseline disease process is difficult and inefficient. In addition, the realities are that most third-party payers will not cover an in-patient stay for the purpose of pulmonary rehabilitation, and that many patients live too far from an outpatient program to make attendance feasible. The purpose of this paper is to present the pluses and minuses of pulmonary rehabilitation during acute hospitalization, and to describe a program that has evolved over the last five years at Duke University Medical Center.

Theresa G. Davidson is Patient Services Coordinator, Department of Physical and Occupational Therapy, Duke University Medical Center, Box 3965, Durham, NC 27710. She was formerly Senior Physical Therapist, Cardiopulmonary Team, at Duke University Medical Center and teaches in the Cardiopulmonary Rehabilitation elective in the Graduate Program in Physical Therapy, Duke University.

31

GOALS/CHALLENGES

There are several goals that can be accomplished via in-patient pulmonary rehabilitation. The first is to improve a patient's understanding of his disease process. The second is to stop the downward spiral of deconditioning that develops with any chronic disease. A third goal is to improve the patient's breathing control through specific breathing exercises and inspiratory muscle training. The final goal is to teach and initiate a comprehensive, progressive exercise program for stretching, strengthening, and endurance training.

Individuals with a chronic disease often become surprisingly accepting of the limitations the disease puts on their lifestyle. This makes it more difficult to find motivational tools (carrots) to increase compliance to something as unappealing as an exercise program. One advantage to beginning pulmonary rehabilitation during the acute hospitalization is that patients are at a "teachable moment." By this we mean that the result of suddenly increased medical symptoms and intervention is a new awareness on the part of the individual of the ravages of his illness; this is accompanied by a resolution to do everything possible to delay or reverse its progress. When patients are at a teachable moment they seem particularly receptive to trying new techniques and are relatively compliant with instructions. They also seem to have good retention of new information while in this frame of mind.

On the other hand, there are several disadvantages to initiating pulmonary rehabilitation during the in-patient stay. The most obvious is that the individual is acutely ill at the time of admission — often with fever, respiratory distress, and increased quantity and tenacity of sputum. In our facility, physical therapy is initiated within twenty-four hours of admission but may consist only of bronchial hygiene (chest physical therapy), breathing exercises, and incentive spirometry for the first two to four days, or until the patient has stabilized. At the latter time, the exercise and education components of the rehabilitation program can be initiated.

Another frustration with attempting pulmonary rehabilitation with the hospitalized patient is the volume of tests for which the patient is scheduled. Some of these (such as x-rays) are a problem only in that physical therapy must be scheduled at other times. Others, such as allergy testing or bronchoscopy, may render the patient unable to exercise for the rest of the day either because of the nature of the procedure or the medications given during it. This problem can be minimized through good communication between nurse and therapist. With advance planning, the patient can be exercised in the early morning before leaving the ward.

The final problem encountered with in-patients is the seemingly endless series of intravenous antibiotics they receive. Certain exercises become impossible in the arm containing the access needle. Also, exercise of the patient away from the ward is difficult if a nurse needs to constantly "fine tune" the flow rate, etc. If these disadvantages are viewed as challenges, rather than road blocks, much still can be achieved through in-patient pulmonary rehabilitation. The groundwork for significant improvements in quality of life and exercise capacity can be established.

EVALUATION

The key to any individualized patient program is an initial evaluation that is comprehensive, repeatable, and, most important, time efficient. There are three main physical areas which should be assessed before beginning pulmonary rehabilitation: strength, flexibility, and endurance. To evaluate strength, a gross test of the large muscle groups is sufficient. In addition to evaluating each muscle against resistance, it is worth noting if the person is able to do ten repetitions without fatiguing. Some pulmonary patients are so debilitated that they will need to stop before completing ten repetitions of any one motion. When evaluating flexibility, extra attention should be given to motion in the rib cage, upper back, shoulders, and neck. As a result of accessory muscle contributions to respiratory effort, these areas can become extremely inflexible.

Endurance can be measured in several different ways. One of the simplest and least expensive is the twelve-minute walk test[2] which can be carried out in any level enclosed hospital corridor. The patient is instructed to cover as much ground as possible within twelve minutes, stopping or changing pace as needed. Blood pressure is measured pre- and post-walking. Heart rate and oxygen saturation are measured continuously with a portable pulse oximeter and the patient uses the same amount of supplemental oxygen as at rest. In patients with chronic bronchitis, this test has been shown to correlate positively with forced vital capacity (FVC) and with maximum oxygen consumption (VO_2) on a bicycle ergometer.[3]

There are two other items that should be evaluated before beginning a pulmonary rehabilitation program. The first of these is the patient's baseline knowledge concerning his disease process and the principles of effective exercise training. Chronically diseased individuals seem to fall all along the continuum of knowledge on these subjects. Some have had their disease for many years and have carefully read and interpreted all the information that is available about their problem. Others are either newly diagnosed or misinformed and lack even the most basic concepts. To be time efficient and to avoid boring the well-informed individual, it is vital to gear the educational component of the program to each person's needs.

The last item to evaluate is the patient's accessibility to resources within his home community. For individuals living within a community with an established out-patient program, home instructions can be kept to a minimum and referral arranged. For patients who will have to be independent with their exercise following discharge from the hospital, access to a stationary ergometer, pool, or indoor track must be determined. Maximum compliance will be achieved if the patient's exercise program prescribed for home use mimics the in-patient hospital program.

PROGRAM COMPONENTS

Once the evaluation is complete, design and implementation of the exercise program can be straightforward. At our facility, the patient is given an empty folder on the first day. Into this all booklets, handouts, and home instruction materials can be placed as they are introduced. An individualized packet is built that can be easily reviewed by other health professionals, family members, and the patient himself.

One of the first things placed in the folder is information on principles of energy conservation. This can be presented even before the individual is ready to begin ambulation. In fact, the more debilitated and short-of-breath the patient, the more earnest is his tendency to assimilate these techniques. Postures for controlling short-ness of breath, techniques for stair climbing (inhale as the leg is lifted and exhale as the body is raised), and avoidance of overhead work are among the most important principles presented. Environ-mental considerations are presented next: (1) avoid activity in high humidity areas (always shower in a well-ventilated bathroom); (2) decrease speed and distance of walking in hot weather; (3)in cold weather, always cover mouth and nose loosely to warm the air be-fore it contacts bronchial passages; and (4) replace all fluids lost in perspiration to avoid dehydration and resultant thickening of bron-chial mucus. If indicated, topics such as breath control during meals,[4] intimacy concerns, and use of nonrestrictive clothing also can be discussed.

Another early facet of the rehabilitation process is breathing exer-cises. Many patients have learned diaphragmatic breathing previ-ously, but do not understand the need to utilize this as their pattern at rest and during activity. Pursed-lip exhalation as a technique for decreasing residual volume (RV) and carbon dioxide levels also is presented. In addition, one of the "tinker toys" of breathing re-training is often introduced early in the rehabilitation sessions. If the individual has difficulty with maximum inspiration, with exhal-ing carbon dioxide sufficiently, or has atelectasis per chest x-ray, an incentive spirometer will be utilized. If the person has the ability to take a single effective breath but has poor respiratory muscle endur-ance, an inspiratory muscle trainer such as the P-flex or Aerobica will be given. In either case, frequent sessions per day are encour-aged.

The final component to pulmonary rehabilitation is the exercise program. At our facility, an attempt is made to style each exercise session like the home program being developed. Thus, each session begins and ends with five to ten minutes of individualized stretching followed by strengthening exercises, forming the warm-up and cool-down at either end of the endurance training component. If the patient is able, the endurance training consists of twenty-five min-utes of walking or stationary ergometry done at an intensity suffi-cient to maintain sixty to eighty percent of tested or age-predicted maximum heart rate. When trained in this manner, the individual with chronic pulmonary disease should be able to reap almost all the benefits associated with aerobic exercise: increased stroke volume, increased arteriovenous oxygen extraction, delayed aerobic threshold and lactic acid production, and reduced minute ventilation (Ve) at each submaximal work level.[5] In most published studies, these individuals have been shown to have no improvements in pulmonary function test results, even with training at an intensity beyond the aerobic threshold.[6]

In reality, the vast majority of patients with chronic obstructive pulmonary disease are unable to train aerobically, especially when hospitalized. In this situation, the goal is to use whatever techniques will allow them to achieve a maximum amount of total training. The theory of specificity of training has become generally accepted: that is, the effect of training will be most pronounced during performance of activity in the mode used for training. Thus, if the patient plans to walk after discharge a walking program is used in the hospital. If he plans to bike at home, similarly a biking program will be initiated. If his work or recreational activities involve a large amount of repetitive upper extremity work, endurance training with the arms can be attempted, although this is particularly difficult for pulmonary patients because of the rib-cage mechanics involved in breathing versus arm work.

When advising patients to choose biking versus walking, several factors may be discussed. Walking is inexpensive and requires no training or equipment. Indoor biking allows exercise without leaving home, without use of a portable oxygen system, at any time of day, and in any kind of weather. Walking can be used as a social outlet while biking is usually a solitary activity. Often one or more of these factors are sufficient to sway a patient toward a particular exercise mode.

If the patient has limited exercise tolerance, a circuit training approach is utilized. We may start with three minute bouts of activity spaced by three minute rests. Gradually, the activity periods are lengthened and the rest periods shortened. The patient is encouraged to rest only until his shortness of breath has decreased to an acceptable level for exercise to resume. When patients have difficulty coordinating breathing patterns with activity, the portable pulse/oximeter may be used as a biofeedback tool. Ninety percent oxygen saturation of the blood is used as an acceptable minimum. The patient practices paced breathing, diaphragmatic breathing and pursed-lip exhalation to see which combination allows more exertion while maintaining at least ninety percent oxygenation. If the patient desaturates despite optimal breathing techniques, supplemental oxygen is added, during endurance exercise only, in 1L/minute increments until an amount is found that prevents desaturation. Oxygen is not administered beyond 4L/minute without specific consent of the physician. Also, care is taken to decrease the amount of supplemental oxygen to the baseline amount immediately upon completion of endurance activity. In patients with carbon dioxide retention, an overabundance of oxygen has the potential to depress the respiratory drive.

Once the basic program is begun, exercise is conducted twice daily, often once with the therapist and once independently by the patient. Duration and intensity are progressed as tolerated and, similarly, education progresses at a level adjusted to the patient's needs. On the final day, the home program is written out, six-week goals and long-term goals are established, and a daily exercise recording log is provided. As with all home programs, the goal is to be comprehensive, yet not complex. Based on subjective assessment of our pulmonary rehabilitation patients seen at a later date, those who follow through post-discharge appear to have greater functional capacity, improved self-image, and slower progression of their disease. Not surprisingly, those most compliant with home exercise are also most compliant with medication, nutrition, and non-smoking instructions.

REFERENCES

1. Pulmonary Rehabilitation: Official American Thoracic Society Statement. Am. Rev. Resp. Dis. 124:663-666, 1981

2. Cooper KN: The New Aerobics. New York, NY, M Evans and Company Inc, 1970, pp 29-30

3. McGavin CR, Gupta SP, McHardy GJ: Twelve minute walking test for assessing disability in chronic bronchitis. Br. Med. J. 1:822-823, 1976

4. Moser KM, Archibald C, Hansen P et al.: Shortness of Breath, A Guide for Better Living and Breathing, ed 3. Toronto, CV Mosby Co, 1983

5. Belman MJ, Wasserman K: Exercise testing and training in patients with chronic obstructive pulmonary disease. Resp. Care 27:724-731, 1982

6. Beuman LB, Sutton JR: Exercise for the pulmonary patient. J. Cardiopulm. Rehab. 6:62-61, 1986

Community-Based Pulmonary Rehabilitation of the Patient with Chronic Obstructive Pulmonary Disease

Rebecca H. Crouch, MS, PT

SUMMARY. In 1984 a community-based pulmonary rehabilitation program was initiated at Duke University Medical Center. A multidisciplinary group planned the program to meet the rehabilitation needs of the pulmonary patient who was not acutely ill. Musculoskeletal and respiratory evaluative procedures were chosen and a comprehensive exercise and pulmonary hygiene program was designed. An individualized treatment regime is planned for the participant who enrolls in each five week course. With approximately 300 patients having completed the Duke program, the need has surfaced to initiate a "graduate program" to provide an organized maintenance exercise routine for those who have been through the intensive rehabilitation course.

INTRODUCTION

Historically, the treatment for persons with Chronic Obstructive Pulmonary Disease (COPD) has been directed toward the remission or stabilization of the acute complications that frequently hospitalize them, or motivate them to seek medical attention. Therapy has focused on treatment of these exacerbations with medications and rest. Once the acute episode subsided, the patients commonly were left on their own to "stay healthy," "do only what you feel like doing, but don't overexert yourself," or "be your own monitor,

Rebecca H. Crouch is Assistant Director, Pulmonary Rehabilitation Program, Duke University Medical Center, P.O. Box 3022, Durham, NC 27710.

your body will tell you when to stop." These clichés may sound good to the health care provider, but they do not provide the individual with pulmonary disease a long-term plan of action to battle his illness.

In the previous article on pulmonary rehabilitation during acute hospitalization, the author discusses inpatient pulmonary rehabilitation currently in place at Duke University Medical Center. The purpose of the present article is to describe the basic components of a community-based pulmonary rehabilitation program that has been in existence in this medical center for the past four years. As the reader will note, these programs have certain goals in common, but also have distinguishing features because of the nature of the patient population and the rehabilitation setting.

DEVELOPMENT OF A COMMUNITY-BASED PULMONARY REHABILITATION PROGRAM

In 1984, a small multidisciplinary group at Duke began to identify the need for an ongoing form of education and therapy for pulmonary patients once they were discharged from the hospital. With the advent of Diagnosis Related Groups (DRGs), many physicians and therapists were frustrated by the lack of time available to rehabilitate pulmonary patients adequately in the hospital setting. Initial gains made while the patient was hospitalized were lost to follow-up care once the patient was discharged. Consequently, we began to design a rehabilitation program with the primary goal of providing exercise and education for the pulmonary patient who was not acutely ill. It was thought that this population would generally "feel better," allowing them to comprehend and practice the techniques of breathing and physical exercise with greater ease.

Several questions were considered by the group responsible for designing the outpatient pulmonary program. Will the program have age, diagnosis, or degree of disability restrictions? What geographical area will the program serve: local, regional, or national? What is the best combination of health care disciplines to employ in a pulmonary rehabilitation program?

Following a one year planning period, the program admitted its first patients in May, 1985. To date, approximately 300 patients have participated. Classes are held in an athletic facility on campus which houses a track, a heated pool, and various exercise equipment. About half of the participants are from North Carolina and the other half primarily are from the eastern United States. Small classes of six to eight patients are scheduled to meet Monday through Friday for four and one-half weeks. The daily schedule begins at 1:00 p.m. and lasts until 5:00 p.m. Afternoons have been chosen for two reasons: (1) in general, people with pulmonary disease have difficulty with breathing, clearing secretions, and activity early in the day, and (2) a four hour daily program allows an efficient use of employee time, permitting the first half of the day to be used by the staff for inpatient care.

Staff members include a pulmonologist as medical director, a biomedical engineer as program director, a physical therapist, and a respiratory therapist. While persons in each discipline have specific duties unique to the profession, many of the day to day tasks can be performed by most of the staff members. The respiratory therapist has been instructed in, and leads, warm-up exercises twice weekly. Likewise, the physical therapist has been instructed in the delivery of bronchodilator treatments. Both perform chest physical therapy.

The Duke Pulmonary Rehabilitation Program has accepted any patient who has expressed an interest in, and motivation to complete, the program, regardless of degree of disability, age, or diagnosis. The program has accepted smokers with certain stipulations: the individual must have a desire to stop smoking and be willing to attend a smoking cessation course. Some patients have been referred by their personal physicians, others have been self-referred, but most have come to the program through word of mouth information from former participants. The program has managed to maintain full enrollment, with waiting lists in the spring and fall as these are particularly desirable times to attend because of favorable weather conditions.

PATIENT EVALUATION AND TREATMENT

The initial patient evaluation includes a symptom limited maximum cycle ergometer exercise test combined with metabolic gas and arterial blood gas analysis, electrocardiogram, and blood pressure monitoring. Static and dynamic pulmonary function tests (PFTs) and a chest x-ray are also obtained prior to entrance into the program.

The initial two days of the program are used for further evaluation and orientation. On the first day of orientation, a 12 minute walk test is performed by all participants on an indoor track where 20 laps are equal to one mile. The physical therapist or respiratory therapist conduct individual interviews with each participant to evaluate the need for aerosol therapy and chest physical therapy. The individual's present activity level is discussed and realistic goals are set by the patient and staff member. Orientation activities also include instruction in breathing exercises and paced-breathing stair climbing. Equipment necessary for the program (pedometers, P-flexes, exercise recording forms, and patient manuals) also are distributed during the orientation period. The patient manual is a compilation of educational lecture outlines, program exercise routines, and equipment information.

The three cornerstones of the program are individualized pulmonary hygiene, progressive exercise, and education. Thirty to forty-five minutes each day are reserved for education. Staff lectures include physiological responses to exercise, inhaler usage, chest anatomy, and functional exercise attire. Guest lecturers from the medical community address psychosocial issues, sexuality, nutrition, pharmacology, and medical ethics. A clinical psychologist, who will join the staff soon, plans to offer counseling in stress management, relaxation, and panic control.

Respiratory therapy consists of daily aerosol therapy and weekly peak flow spirometry. Both the physical therapist and the respiratory therapist perform chest physical therapy after bronchodilator therapy and instruct the patients in breathing exercises.

ROLE OF THE PHYSICAL THERAPIST

The role of the physical therapist in the pulmonary rehabilitation program is two-fold: (1) to evaluate the cardiopulmonary status of the patient and to provide the treatment indicated, and (2) to evaluate the musculoskeletal system and to design an appropriate exercise program.

Cardiopulmonary Evaluation and Treatment

The physical therapist evaluates the patient's present cardiopulmonary status and establishes a current and long-term treatment plan. Recent chest x-rays, arterial blood gases, PFTs, and medications, including oxygen, are assessed. At the time of the examination and interview, breath sounds, current history of sputum production, body temperature, and breathing pattern are evaluated. Palpation of the chest wall and accessory breathing muscles, as well as a review of the PFTs (particularly the maximum voluntary ventilation) and observation of the breathing pattern, help determine the strength and endurance of the diaphragm and intercostal muscles. The patient also is asked about home therapy. What equipment does he have? Is he following a particular schedule of breathing treatments and chest physical therapy? Is the patient able to administer treatments to himself, or does he require help from a family member? How well does the regime work?

Based on the results of this evaluation, a treatment plan and goals are established. The treatment plan may include any or all of the following: aerosol therapy followed by chest physical therapy (postural drainage, percussion, and vibration), instruction of the patient and family members in chest physical therapy, and ordering necessary equipment for home care (an air compressor for bronchodilator delivery, mechanical percussor, or portable oxygen). In addition, diaphragmatic and pursed-lip breathing exercises are included in the treatment program, with emphasis upon coordinating rhythmic breathing with exercise. Patients are instructed to use these breathing patterns in different positions, to exhale during the most difficult phase of any activity, and NEVER to hold their breath.

Another important facet of pulmonary care includes inspiratory muscle training. A P-flex may be used to strengthen the muscles of inspiration and increase their endurance.[1] Patients are instructed to begin training for 15 minutes twice daily and increase the degree of breathing resistance weekly while keeping the duration and respiratory rate constant.

Musculoskeletal Evaluation and Treatment

The second major role of the physical therapist is to conduct a musculoskeletal evaluation and design an exercise treatment program. A comprehensive exercise program for pulmonary patients includes three components: (1) aerobic, (2) anaerobic, and (3) relaxation exercises.

Aerobic activities include exercises in which large muscle groups are used in rhythmic contractions. Following the principle of specificity of exercise, the patient is trained in a modality of exercise that will be useful in daily living. Walking exercise therefore is valuable because it is needed to perform most daily activities. Bicycling, using a stationery bike or a Schwinn Airdyne, is a modality that improves the strength and coordination of lower extremity musculature. Arm ergometry, using an Airdyne or Cybex Upper Body Exerciser, can improve the function of upper extremity and shoulder girdle musculature.

During aerobic activities, special attention must be given to the patient's oxygen saturation. Finger or ear oximetry provides valuable information about the patient's need for supplemental oxygen during exercise. In the Duke outpatient program, an oxygen saturation of 88% or below has been chosen by the medical director as the point at which supplemental oxygen should be used. The Borg Scale of Perceived Exertion is a useful tool in the assessment of the degree of difficulty of particular tasks for the pulmonary patient. Even though a target heart rate is probably not necessary in the COPD population, some attention must be given to the work of the heart with exercise. Patients who perform work near their maximum heart rate over a period of minutes do become quite fatigued and are probably exerting maximum effort.[2]

Anaerobic exercises are valuable for improving strength and flexibility of muscles and joints. Cuff weights, dumbbells, Theraband, and Nautilus are useful modalities to strengthen muscles. Flexibility exercises should target typical problem areas for the COPD population, namely the hamstrings, gastrocnemii, pectorals, and low back extensors. Faulty postural habits are common among pulmonary patients and require special consideration. Exercises are necessary to improve chest wall mobility and to correct the typical forward head and rounded shoulders posture seen in these patients.

Other anaerobic activities that can complement a comprehensive rehabilitation program are stair climbing, pool exercise, and backpack walking.[3] Even though these modalities can be used in aerobic training, the emphasis for pulmonary patients is placed on slowing the pace, coordinating breathing, and strengthening muscles.

Relaxation exercises may be added to a COPD rehabilitation program. Chronically elevated and tense upper trapezii muscles are common among pulmonary patients. Biofeedback has been found to be useful in increasing patients' awareness of tension and has helped them progressively relax these muscles. Jacobson's relaxation exercises, massage, and imagery also are tools that assist with patient relaxation.

DOCUMENTATION AND REFERRAL

Staff members of the Duke rehabilitation program have found it to be extremely important to document the patient's evaluation and progress. Because of the large number of participants who are under Medicare coverage, care must be taken to obtain physician referrals and write thorough evaluation, progress, and discharge notes. Members of each discipline document according to specific Medicare guidelines for outpatient rehabilitation.

The location of the outpatient rehabilitation program in a medical center setting has its advantages for availability of referral resources. Duke has a stop-smoking program that we strongly urge all smoking participants to attend. Cardiologists and other specialty physicians are available for consultation should the need arise. Some of the participants with special nutritional needs consult with a dietician for the duration of the program. Others may be referred to the biofeedback laboratory for anxiety and panic control.

"GRADUATION" ACTIVITIES

Graduation from the program is a big event, complete with diplomas, T-shirts, and a pot luck party on the last day. In addition, all participants have a discharge cycle ergometer exercise test, PFTs, and a 12 minute walk. They take home with them an individualized exercise and walking program as well as a two month diary for recording daily walking, P-flex, and exercise sessions. Audio and videocassettes of the floor exercise routine are made available to the participants; these have been particularly successful in improving compliance with home exercise. Because many of the patients live some distance away from the medical center, a newsletter is published quarterly to update graduates on medication, equipment, and newsy items pertaining to the program, its staff, and participants.

The staff views outpatient pulmonary rehabilitation as an opportunity to allow and encourage our patients to have fun and feel successful in addition to giving them an opportunity to improve their physical condition. Although a great deal of hard work is required to "graduate," most of the patients are proud that they were able to accomplish activities that they would not have considered doing only five weeks ago.

FUTURE PLANS

Future plans for the Duke University Medical Center outpatient pulmonary rehabilitation program include a "graduate program" for those who have been through the intensive program and who live nearby. The graduate program will include expanded aerobic and strength training activities such as rowing, Stairmaster, and pool aerobics.

REFERENCES

1. Sonne LJ, Davis JA: Increased exercise performance in patients with severe COPD following inspiratory resistive training. Chest 81: 436-439, 1982

2. Belman MJ, Wasserman K: Exercise training and testing in patients with chronic obstructive pulmonary disease. Respiratory Care 27: 724-731, 1982

3. Abstract from the International Conference on Pulmonary Rehabilitation and Home Mechanical Ventilation March 1988: O'Hara WJ, Lasachuk KE: Anaerobic training advantages in COPD. Department of Respirology, St. Joseph's Health Center, Toronto, Canada

In-Patient Rehabilitation of the Coronary Artery Bypass Surgery Patient and the Heart Transplantation Patient

Andrea R. DeArmott, PT

SUMMARY. Cardiac rehabilitation is a comprehensive approach to patient care that includes physical therapy, nursing, social services, discharge planning assistance, and chaplain services. The rehabilitative process begins early after surgery. Rehabilitation is progressive and consists of aerobic activity, range of motion exercise, chest physical therapy and patient education. The author provides an overview of the physical therapy intervention required by the coronary artery bypass surgery patient and the heart transplantation patient.

INTRODUCTION

Cardiac rehabilitation is an ongoing multidisciplinary intervention. The goal is to restore cardiac patients to their optimal levels of physical, psychological, social, and vocational function.[1] This article will focus on the in-hospital cardiac rehabilitation provided by physical therapists for patients recovering from coronary artery bypass graft surgery (CABGS) and heart transplantation (HT) at Duke University Medical Center.

The in-patient cardiac rehabilitation is intended to help alleviate problems associated with bedrest, reduce anxiety, reduce depression, develop the patient's confidence, provide education, increase

---

At the time this article was written, Andrea R. DeArmott was Senior Physical Therapist, Cardiopulmonary Rehabilitation, Department of Physical Therapy, Duke University Medical Center, Durham, NC 27710.

47

the chance of timely hospital discharge and return to work, and provide surveillance for optimal patient management.[2]

CRITERIA FOR ENTRY INTO THE CARDIAC REHABILITATION PROGRAM

Patients enter the cardiac rehabilitation program by referral of their cardiac surgeon. In general, the postoperative cardiac patient who is clinically stable and infection-free may safely begin the progressive activity portion of the in-patient cardiac rehabilitation program perhaps as early as 24 hours after surgery. Contraindications and considerations for entry into the progressive activity program follow.[2,14]

Absolute Contraindications

1. Patients on bedrest with motion restrictions
2. Prolonged or unstable angina pectoris
3. Recent acute myocardial infarction (MI) with unstable condition
4. Resting diastolic blood pressure (BP) over 120 mm Hg or resting systolic blood pressure over 200 mm Hg
5. Inappropriate blood pressure response: a symptomatic orthostatic or exercise-induced drop in systolic blood pressure of 10 to 20 mm Hg
6. Severe atrial or ventricular dysrhythmias
7. Second or third-degree heart block
8. Recent embolism, either systemic or pulmonary
9. Thrombophlebitis
10. Dissecting aneurysm
11. Fever greater than 100 degrees F: for the patient in the critical-care area, 102 degrees F
12. Excessive sternal movement (contraindication for upper extremity and trunk range of motion [ROM] exercises)
13. Uncompensated heart failure
14. Active pericarditis (primary) or myocarditis
15. Severe aortic stenosis (more than 50 mm Hg gradient)
16. Acute systemic illness

Relative Contraindications

1. Resting diastolic blood pressure over 110 mm Hg or resting systolic blood pressure over 180 mm Hg
2. Inappropriate increase in blood pressure with exercise (systolic blood pressure greater than or equal to 220 mm Hg or diastolic blood pressure greater than or equal to 110 mm Hg)
3. Hypotension (less than 90/60 mm Hg)
4. Asymptomatic orthostatic drop of 10 to 20 mm Hg in systolic blood pressure
5. Moderate aortic stenosis (25 mm Hg to 50 mm Hg gradient)
6. Compensated heart failure
7. Significant emotional stress
8. Pericarditis associated with myocardial revascularization surgery
9. Resting ST-segment depression (greater than 3 mm)
10. Uncontrolled diabetes
11. Neuromuscular, musculoskeletal, or arthritic disorders that would prevent activity
12. Excessive incisional drainage
13. Sinus tachycardia greater than 120 beats/minute at rest
14. Postoperative or post-MI electrocardiographic (ECG) changes indicative or suggestive of fresh infarct
15. Ventricular aneurysm
16. Symptomatic anemia (hematocrit less than 30 percent)

Conditions Requiring Special Consideration and Precaution

1. Conduction disturbances: left bundle branch block, Wolff-Parkinson-White Syndrome, and Lown Ganong-Levine Syndrome
2. Controlled dysrhythmias
3. Fixed-rate pacemaker
4. Mitral valve prolapse
5. Angina pectoris and other manifestations of coronary insufficiency
6. Electrolyte disturbance
7. Cyanotic heart disease

8. Marked obesity (20 percent above desirable body weight)
9. Renal, hepatic, or other metabolic insufficiency
10. Moderate to severe pulmonary disease
12. Intermittent claudication

REHABILITATION AFTER CORONARY ARTERY BYPASS GRAFT SURGERY

Evaluation

It is important to note that a complete patient evaluation should be performed prior to the initiation of physical therapy. The evaluation includes the past medical history; the history of present illness; pre and postoperative activity level; the type of surgery and date performed; complications with surgery; evaluation of pulmonary status, i.e., auscultation, breathing pattern, cough and sputum production; a review of tests, i.e., chest x-ray, arterial blood gases, and cardiac/pulmonary function tests; lines in situ; medications; vital signs; initial exercise evaluation; and chart documentation.

Aerobic Exercise

Individualized prescriptive exercise is the hallmark of rehabilitative physical activity and has been shown to be feasible and safe for appropriately selected patients (see previous list of contraindications). The prescriptive components of rehabilitative physical activity include the frequency, duration, and intensity of exercise and the type of exercise to be undertaken.[5] In some institutions, the activity component of the rehabilitation program is initiated as early as 24 hours after surgery. Early mobilization has been shown to help offset the adverse effects of bedrest.[3,4]

Moderate ambulation at a low intensity (1 to 2 METS)* begins at distances of 100-300 feet 2 times a day. Note that a speed of 1 to 2 METS equals less than or equal to 1.5 to 2 miles per hour.[14] Ambulation is increased by distance and frequency as the patient tolerates. The *time* it takes the patient to cover the distance during ambu-

---

1 MET or metabolic unit = 3.5 ml O_2/kg body weight/minute

lation should be recorded since this parameter will be used when designing the patient's home aerobic program. Biking can be substituted for ambulation as the aerobic portion of the patient's program. The time spent cycling should equal the time spent ambulating and should be done with the resistance set on zero.[6] The patient should cycle at a RPM (revolutions per minute) speed that reproduces the ambulation speed of less than or equal to 1.5 to 2 miles per hour.[14]

Heart rate, blood pressure and the Rating of Perceived Exertion (RPE) are utilized to provide information on the patient's hemodynamics and aerobic exercise tolerance, and to progress the patient through the in-patient rehabilitation program.

Patients who are receiving betablocking or calcium channel blocking drugs as part of their medication regime should be observed closely during exercise. Their heart rate and blood pressure may not respond appropriately to increased oxygen demand, and the patients may not complain of fatigue despite the activity level. In this patient population, the scale of perceived exertion should be used to better evaluate the patient's response to activity.[12]

Heart rate, blood pressure, and RPE are evaluated at rest, after aerobic exercise, and 5 minutes after termination of aerobic exercise. As noted previously, early in-patient exercise is usually conducted within a 2 MET level.[2] The upper-limit training/target heart rate (THR) is 20 beats/minute above the standing resting heart rate. A RPE level of 11 to 12 is felt to be appropriate during the in-patient phase—a rating of 13 (somewhat hard) on the RPE scale corresponds to 20 beats/minute above the standing resting heart rate.[7] Unless a predischarge graded exercise test (GXT) is performed, these standards apply until a symptom-limited graded exercise test (SL-GXT) is performed at 4 to 8 weeks after surgery.[2,8]

The careful monitoring of intensity is important to overall safety in the exercise training of cardiac patients. During the first 6 to 8 weeks of training, progression is achieved mainly through increased duration and frequency of training and, to a lesser extent, through increasing intensity. Significant cardiac events i.e., arrhythmias, myocardial ischemia or infarct, have been shown to be more related to intensity of exercise rather than to either frequency or duration of training.[9,10]

The cardiac rehabilitation practitioner should be aware of the following indications to modify or terminate the exercise routine:[8,11]

1. Fatigue
2. Failure of monitoring equipment
3. Lightheadedness, confusion, ataxia, pallor, cyanosis, dyspnea, nausea, or any peripheral circulatory insufficiency
4. Onset of angina with exercise
5. Symptomatic supraventricular tachycardia
6. ST-segment displacement greater than 2 mm horizontal or downsloping from rest
7. Ventricular tachycardia (three or more consecutive premature ventricular contractions [PVCs])
8. Exercise-induced left or right bundle branch block
9. Onset of second- and third-degree heart block
10. One R on T PVC
11. Frequent unifocal PVCs (more than 10/minute)
12. Frequent multifocal PVCs (more than 10/minute)
13. PVC couplets (more than 2/minute)
14. Increase in heart rate of more than 20 beats/minute above standing resting rate
15. Drop of greater than or equal to 10 mm Hg in systolic blood pressure
16. Excessive blood-pressure rise: systolic greater than or equal to 220 mm Hg or diastolic greater than or equal to 120 mm Hg
17. Inappropriate bradycardia (drop in heart rate greater than 10 beats/minute) with increase or no change in workload
18. Drop of greater than or equal to 10 mm Hg in diastolic blood pressure

Goals for the aerobic exercise at discharge include frequent (2 to 3 times/day) ambulation or cycling for 5 to 10 minutes at a low intensity of 1.2 to 2.5 METS. Patients can safely increase their aerobic activity by 5 minutes each week. During the next six to eight weeks, the duration of aerobic exercise increases to 20 to 30 minutes at a moderate intensity of 2 to 3 METS and the frequency decreases to 1 to 2 times/day.[6]

Proper warm-up and cool-down phases prior to and after the aerobic portion of the exercise program are essential. In addition to preparing the body for the upcoming workout, the warm-up is a precaution against unnecessary injuries and muscle soreness. The warm-up progressively stimulates the heart and lungs, increases the blood flow, and gradually increases the temperature of the blood and muscles. A complete warm-up lasts 5 to 10 minutes and will stretch the muscles and tendons in preparation for more forceful contractions. The cool-down is a tapering-off period after completion of the main workout. It is best accomplished by a continuation of activity at a lowered intensity level. During the cool-down period it is best to repeat the stretching exercises used before the aerobic portion of the workout. Generally, a 5 to 10 minute recovery period is sufficient.[14]

Since most patients encounter stairs either at home or in daily activities, stair climbing is a regular component of the progressive activity program. Dion et al.[3] found that hypotension, as defined by an exercise-induced drop in the systolic blood pressure of more than 10 mm Hg, occurred more often after stair climbing than after treadmill ambulation or range of motion exercises; therefore, it is recommended that patients be closely supervised while performing stair-climbing activities.

Patients are usually discharged from the hospital 7 to 10 days after surgery providing there are no delaying complications.

Range of Motion Exercises

The CABGS patient sustains significant soft tissue and bone damage of the chest wall during the surgical procedure. If this area does not receive ROM exercise, adhesions may develop and the musculature can become weaker and contractures can develop. Patients also will favor the arm, shoulder and chest areas, which tends to result in poor posture and which makes the attainment of previous strength and full ROM more difficult. Patients who experience sternal movement or have postsurgical wound complications should not perform these exercises.[6]

The arm ROM exercises include bilateral shoulder flexion, extension, abduction, and shoulder elevation within the range of the patient's comfort. Horizontal abduction beyond the frontal plane is avoided to prevent excessive tension on the healing sternum. Initially leg ROM exercises include hip flexion and extension with knee flexion and extension, hip abduction and adduction, internal and external rotation, and ankle plantar-flexion, dorsiflexion, inversion and eversion.[2]

Range of motion exercises should continue for 6 to 8 weeks postoperatively. During this time, clinical boney union of the sternum occurs along with soft tissue healing.[2] Studies have shown that minimal to mild stress to the healing boney structures optimizes the healing process.[13]

As the patient is able to ambulate longer distances and discharge from the hospital nears, he should be instructed in arm, trunk, and leg "stretches" to be used for the warm-up and cool-down phases in conjunction with slow aerobic activity. The arm stretches used should include (but not be limited to) full shoulder flexion, abduction, and circumduction. Trunk stretches include lateral flexion without rotation, and gentle flexion and extension. Many leg stretches are available to the patient; however, the muscles that need to be stretched prior to and after aerobic exercise include the hip flexors (iliopsoas and rectus femoris), quadriceps muscle group, hamstring muscle group, and the gastrocnemius-soleus muscle group.

Chest Physical Therapy

The purpose of chest physical therapy (CPT), also known as bronchial hygiene, is to assist the clearance of pulmonary secretions. Techniques include postural drainage, manual or mechanical percussion and vibration, and instruction in coughing and breathing exercises.

In the postoperative cardiac patient, there may be any number of reasons why the patient requires CPT. These include (1) increased body temperature secondary to decreased inspiratory effort and/or mucous plugging causing atelectasis; (2) abnormal chest x-ray except with the presence of a pleural effusion; (3) presence of adventitious breath sounds; or (4) increased secretion retention secondary to underlying chronic lung disease.[15]

There are specific contraindications and precautions for CPT treatment.[15] Contraindications are:

1. Acute pneumothorax and/or flail chest
2. Acute pulmonary embolism
3. Acute cardiac disease i.e., evolving MI
4. Platelet count of less than or equal to 30,000/mm^3

Precautions (requiring modification of treatment) are:

1. Greater than 20 cc hemoptysis — physician should be consulted regarding continuation of CPT
2. Gastroesophageal reflux — the patient may not be able to lie flat
3. Increased intracranial pressure will require position modification
4. Osteoporosis — the treated area should be cushioned with a towel during percussion and vibration
5. Incisions/chest tubes are never percussed
6. Fractured ribs, in the absence of flail chest, are not percussed for 6 weeks
7. Percussion or vibration should not be done anteriorly in the region of the sternotomy incision, as this may cause microinjury to the sternum and hinder healing.[13,15]

Patient Education

Education and counseling of cardiac patients and their families provides the information and skills that enable them to assume much responsibility for the home cardiac rehabilitation program. This education should include an individualized progressive aerobic exercise program with warm-up and cool-down periods, ROM exercises, exercise guidelines regarding why, where, when and what to wear, basic activity guidelines to avoid sternal healing complications (i.e., no lifting greater than 10 pounds for 6 weeks,[13]) instruction in both radial pulse-taking and use of the RPE scale, and risk factor modification. *Written* directions should be provided to minimize conflicts between the patient and family that may derive from vague or ambiguous recommendations and instructions.[5]

Since cardiac rehabilitation is a multidisciplinary team effort, nursing, dietary, social services, discharge planning assistance and chaplain services should be available and offered to the patient in order to provide comprehensive patient care.

REHABILITATION AFTER HEART TRANSPLANTATION

Introduction

In the past few years heart transplantation has become a more common and accepted treatment for carefully selected patients with endstage heart failure, an abnormality that results in the inability of the heart to supply oxygen at a rate demanded by the metabolizing tissues.[16] Since the introduction of cyclosporine A in 1980, which shows promise of reducing rejection, many centers that had discontinued performing this surgery are once again performing heart transplantations.[17] Potential candidates for cardiac transplantation typically present with low exercise tolerance, cachexia with generalized weakness and decreased muscle mass, marginal blood pressure, dyspnea, and poor peripheral perfusion. Orthopnea, ascites, and peripheral edema are seen in biventricular failure. The quality of the lives of these individuals is severely compromised.[16] Physical therapists are involved in the rehabilitation of these patients both pre and post-operatively. In this discussion of postoperative rehabilitation, characteristics of the function of the normal versus the transplanted heart, special considerations of the heart transplant patient, and the physical therapy intervention including exercise and education will be stressed.

Exercise Response

Prior to discussion of the denervated transplanted heart's response to exercise it is necessary briefly to review the action of the normal innervated heart.

The force of cardiac muscle contraction and the heart rate, in normally innervated heart, are increased by direct stimulation of the sympathetic nervous system. Additionally, stimulation of the adrenal medullae causes release of the catecholamine hormones epinephrine and norepinephrine. Eighty percent of the hormone released is epinephrine, which increases the strength and rate of cardiac muscle contractility. Norepinephrine increases the total peripheral resistance and has less effect on cardiac output. The heart can still function effectively if one of the two mechanisms, i.e., direct sympathetic stimulation and hormonal stimulation, is missing. This dual method of stimulation acts as a safety mechanism in case one of the two is unable to function. Since the recipient's autonomic nervous system is not connected to the donor heart during surgery, the transplanted heart is denervated; therefore, only the hormonal stimulation limb is still intact.[18,19,20]

The denervated heart at rest generally has a higher than normal heart rate. This increased heart rate is a result of lack of vagal stimulation of the donor sinus node. The heart rate in the cardiac transplant population is not affected by the Valsalva maneuver or carotid sinus massage (normally these actions would reduce heart rate). No appreciable change occurs in the heart rate of the cardiac transplant recipient when moving from supine to standing or after receiving atropine (normally these actions would also increase heart rate). Cardiac output, stroke volume, and respiratory rate remain within normal limits in the transplanted heart patient at rest, although it is thought that the cardiac output is slightly lower than that of an individual whose heart is innervated.[21,22,23]

In the normal population, during dynamic exercise heart rate increases immediately in a linear fashion and is mainly responsible for the increase in cardiac output seen early in exercise. Stroke volume, in the normal heart, stays about the same until more strenuous exercise occurs and then increases according to the Frank Starling law, causing an additional increase in cardiac output.[24]

In the cardiac transplant recipient, heart rate starts higher, increases gradually over time (because of circulating catecholamines from the adrenal medullae) and does not reach normal peak heart rate values. Starling's law is thought to be the explanation for the initially observed increase in stroke volume, because more blood is being returned to the heart by the peripheral exercising muscles.

The heart muscle contraction is therefore more forceful, and an increase in stroke volume results. As intensity of exercise increases, further increases in stroke volume occur as a result of the chronotropic and inotropic actions of circulating catecholamines. The result of the catecholamines is an increase in cardiac output. Nonetheless, cardiac output at peak exercise has been shown to be slightly less than that of normals.[24]

During the recovery period following exercise, the normal heart quickly accommodates to the decrease in the intensity of activity by decreasing its rate. In the denervated heart, heart rate decreases more gradually since re-uptake of the circulating catecholamines is slow. In both the innervated and denervated heart, stroke volume promptly begins to decrease after exercise because preload is decreased. The denervated heart, however, may not accommodate to resting values as quickly as the innervated heart.[21,22,23]

With isometric exercise, a similar increase in systolic and diastolic blood pressure occurs in normals and transplant recipients. An increase in total peripheral resistance rather than an increase in cardiac output is responsible for this response. No significant increase in stroke volume occurs in either population. Heart rate reflexively increases in the normal population while no heart rate change is seen in the transplant population.[23,25,26,27]

Special Considerations

Several of the medications that transplant patients require to prevent graft rejection and atherosclerotic changes may cause resting hypertension. These include cyclosporine A, sodium methylprednisolone succinate (Solu Medrol) and prednisone.[17]

Since the transplanted heart is denervated, the patient is unable to perceive the pain associated with myocardial ischemia that may accompany atherosclerosis of the coronary arteries.[16]

Psychologically, the heart transplant time is a period of intense emotion. This emotion is coupled with a sense of well-being as the patient and family celebrate the gift of life and develop an optimistic outlook toward resuming independent, normal living. Transplant recipients are usually highly motivated and eager to learn and progress.[16]

Physical Therapy Intervention

Evaluation

As with the CABGS patient it is important that a complete patient evaluation be performed prior to the initiation of physical therapy. (Refer to the previous section on "Evaluation.")

Intensive Care Unit

Heart transplant patients receive a five day regimen of Antithymocyte Globulin (rabbit origin — rATG) starting immediately postoperatively. The rATG is part of the immunosuppressive regimen. Therapeutic ultrasound treatments to the area of injection follow each rATG injection and they may continue one to three days after the rATG protocol has been completed depending on the extent of the inflammatory reaction to the rATG.[17] The goals of ultrasound are to reduce pain, reduce muscle spasm, and stimulate local blood flow to assist in mobilizing inflammatory infiltrates and edema.[33] Parameters for treatment are (1) intensity at 1.5 w/cm2; (2) duration of 4 minutes at the continuous setting followed by 4 minutes at the pulsed setting; and (3) area to receive ultrasound includes all injection sites (usually located in the vastus lateralis muscle bilaterally). Normal ultrasound gel is used. All isolation precautions as outlined by the hospital should be observed including the proper cleaning of any equipment brought into the patient's room. Light circular massage over the quadriceps muscle for 2-4 minutes after the ultrasound and range of motion exercises may be beneficial in mobilizing any accumulations of fluid and stretching adhesions between muscle fibers brought on by inflammation from the rATG serum.[28]

In addition to the ultrasound treatment, the patient receives gentle passive range of motion exercise to both legs: hip flexion and extension with knee flexion and extension, hip abduction and adduction, hip internal and external rotation, and ankle plantarflexion, dorsiflexion, inversion, and eversion. These ROM exercises will help minimize muscle tightness and venous stasis secondary to immobility and pain.

Depending on his medical/hemodynamic stability, the patient begins active-assisted exercises, progressing to active arm and leg exercises. The leg exercises have been described previously. The arm exercises include bilateral shoulder flexion and extension, shoulder abduction and shoulder elevation within the patient's comfort. These range of motion exercises are necessary to avoid muscle shortening in the shoulder girdle musculature, and are done bilaterally to avoid shifting of the sternum and to allow normal healing to occur. Active exercises of neck rotation, flexion, extension and lateral flexion may be started. In the intensive care unit (ICU), care must be taken to avoid shoulder flexion and abduction beyond 90 degrees if the patient has a Swan-Ganz catheter in position, as movement may move the balloon tip out of position.[29]

By the seventh day postoperatively, much of the patient's initial fatigue and lethargy have resolved and he will tolerate bed to chair ambulation, reclining in the chair, and participating in bedside self-care.[16] By the seventh to ninth day, the patient is moved from the ICU to the ward where isolation precautions continue to be observed.

Rehabilitation on the Ward

Aerobic Exercise

Patients begin a low-level ambulation and/or biking program after transfer to the ward. Both blood pressure and heart rate are monitored at rest, after the warm-up period, after the aerobic exercise, and after the cool-down period. The RPE scale is used in conjunction with the vital signs previously mentioned primarily because of the delayed response of the heart rate to exercise.[30]

Initially, the duration of the activity depends on the patient's tolerance, typically beginning at 5 minutes without resistance on the bike, or at a slow pace while ambulating. Duration progresses to at least 15 minutes of aerobic exercise. When this level is easily tolerated on the bike, resistance is increased. Initial resistance is at 1.4 kpm for 5 minutes and increased by 1/4 kpm after the patient can tolerate 15 minutes of resisted cycling.[15] The ultimate resistance achieved by the patient is individual, but should not exceed the maximum workload of any Exercise Tolerance Test (ETT) performed by the cardiologist. The goal with biking would be to attain

20-30 minutes of continuous cycling at a RPE level of 13-15 or at a training heart rate range as determined by the ETT.[14]

The ambulation program progresses in duration and pace as tolerated. After comfortably walking a 1/4 mile, stairs are begun. The goal by discharge is to attain an endurance level of one continuous mile or 20-30 minutes of continuous ambulation and 1-2 flights of stairs in a reciprocal pattern.[16]

All aerobic activity is preceded by a 10 minute warm-up and followed by a 10 to 15 minute cool-down. The rationale for an extended warm-up in the HT patient is to allow the circulating catecholamines to stimulate heart rate, increase stroke volume, and increase cardiac output to provide oxygen for the metabolizing tissues during the aerobic activity.[31] A long cool-down period is necessary to allow the removal of these hormones by the process of re-uptake into the nerve endings.[18]

The muscles and tendons of the arms, trunk and legs should be stretched to prevent injury during the more vigorous aerobic activity. Stretching is equally important after vigorous activity as a precaution against unnecessary muscle soreness.[14] Stretches, as described in the ROM exercise section of the CABGS rehabilitation portion of this article, are also appropriate for HT patients during the warm-up and cool-down phases.

The Borg RPE scale should be used to determine exertional levels during aerobic activity. Level 6 is a normal resting state and maximal exertion should not exceed level 13-15.[32] The target heart rate (THR) for aerobic training can best be calculated to be half the difference between peak and resting heart rates added to the resting rate. The formula is below:[16]

$$THR = [PHR - RHR/2] + RHR$$

The peak heart rate values are determined from an ETT.[16]

Range of Motion Exercises/Body Mechanics

Heart transplantation patients sustain the same type of soft tissue and bone damage of the chest wall as CABGS patients and require the same type of arm ROM exercises for the same reasons as previously described.

Generally speaking, HT patients remain in the hospital for 3 to 4 weeks. Therefore, they have the opportunity to work on strengthening their arm muscles in addition to working on promoting normal flexibility.

The patient continues performing 10 to 20 repetitions of bilateral arm exercises daily. Sitting extremity exercises are gradually progressed to light resistance with 1 to 2 pounds. Proximal arm workload depends on sternal comfort and healing and is usually limited to a maximum of 3 to 4 pounds. Tolerance for distal resistance is often greater depending on the preoperative status and is limited to 10 pounds during the first 6 to 8 weeks postoperatively.

Preventative back care is emphasized in view of the frequent later side effects of steroids that contribute to osteoporosis, pain, and compression fractures. Patients are instructed in postural awareness, alignment, and optimal body mechanics.[16]

Chest Physical Therapy

The same guidelines for CPT in the CABGS patient apply to the HT patient. Please refer to that section for information.

Patient Education

In addition to the basic education (e.g., activity guidelines, home exercise program) provided to the CABGS patient, the HT patient needs to understand the special exercise responses of the denervated heart. He should realize that this exercise program is designed to provide the tools to maximize his aerobic capacity and strength and, in turn, allow him to function at optimal levels.

REFERENCES

1. Hellerstein HK, Ford AB: Rehabilitation of the cardiac patient. JAMA 164: 225-231, 1957

2. Pollock ML, Pels AE, Foster C, Ward A: Exercise prescription for rehabilitation of the cardiac patient. Pollock ML, Schmidt DH, (eds); Heart Disease and Rehabilitation, ed 2. New York, John Wiley, 1986, pp 447-516

3. Dion FW, Grevenow P, Pollock ML, Squires RW, Foster C, Johnson WD, Schmidt DH: Medical problems and physiologic responses during super-

vised inpatient cardiac rehabilitation: The patient after coronary bypass grafting. Heart Lung 11: 248-255, 1982

4. Silvidi GE, Squires RW, Pollock ML, Foster C: Hemodynamic responses and medical problems associated with early exercise and ambulation in coronary artery bypass surgery patients. J Cardiac Rehabil 65: 134-140, 1982

5. Wenger NK: Rehabilitation of the coronary patient: Status 1986. Progress Cardiovasc Diseases 3: 181-204, 1986

6. Metier CP, Pollock ML, Graves JE: Exercise prescription for the coronary artery bypass graft surgery patient. J. Cardiopul Rehabil 6: 85-103, 1986

7. Rod JL, Squires RW, Pollock ML, Foster C, Schmidt DH: Symptom-limited graded exercise testing soon after myocardial revascularization surgery. J Cardiac Rehabil 2: 199-205, 1982

8. Pollock ML, Wilmore JH, Fox SM: Exercise in health and disease: Evaluation and prescription for prevention and rehabilitation. Philadelphia, WB Saunders, 1984

9. Haskell WL: Cardiovascular complications during training of cardiac patients. Circulation 57: 920-924, 1974

10. Hossack KF, Hartwig R: Cardiac arrest associated with supervised cardiac rehabilitation. J Cardiac Rehabil 2: 402-405, 1982

11. American College of Sports Medicine: Guidelines for Graded Exercise Testing and Exercise Prescription, ed 3. Philadelphia, Lea & Febiger, 1986

12. Williams MA: Principles and methods of exercise testing. In Fardy PS, Bennett JL, Reitz NC, Williams MA (eds): Cardiac Rehabilitation: Implications for the Nurse and Other Health Professionals. St. Louis, CV Mosby, 1980, pp 52-72

13. Nordin M, Frankel VH: Biomechanics of whole bones and bone tissue. In Franbee VH, Norden M (eds): Basic Biomechanics of the Skeletal System. Philadelphia, Lea & Febiger, 1980, pp 15-57

14. Strauss RH: Sportsmedicine. Philadelphia, WB Saunders, 1984

15. Perlstein MF: Cardiovascular and Thoracic Surgery. In Frownfelter DL (ed): Chest Physical Therapy and Pulmonary Rehabilitation — An Interdisciplinary Approach. Chicago, Year Book Medical Publishers, 1978, pp 217-222, 249-266

16. Arthur EK: Rehabilitation of potential and cardiac transplant recipients. APTA Cardiopulm Section Journal, Winter, 1986, pp 11-13

17. Sadowsky HS: The immune system and immunosuppression. APTA Cardiopulm Section Journal, Winter, 1986, pp 2-6

18. Guyton A: Structure and Function of the Nervous System. Philadelphia, WB Saunders, 1976

19. Barr M: The Human Nervous System. New York, Harper & Row, 1979

20. Vander A, Sherman J, Luciano D: Human Physiology — The Mechanisms of Body Function. New York, McGraw-Hill, 1975

21. Leachman R, Leatherman L, Rochelle D et al.: Physiologic behavior of the transplanted heart in six human recipients. Am J Cardiol 23: 123-124, 1969

22. Hammond H, Froelicher V: Normal and abnormal heart rate responses to exercise. Progress Cardiovasc Disease 27: 271-296, 1985

23. Cooper D, Lanza R: Heart Transplantation: The Present Status of Orthotopic and Heterotopic Transplantation. Lancaster, England, MTP Limited, 1984, pp 305-319

24. Guyton A: Textbook of Medical Physiology. Philadelphia, WB Saunders, 1976

25. Savin W, Haskell W, Schroeder F et al.: Cardiorespiratory responses of cardiac transplant patients to graded, symptom-limited exercise. Circulation 62: 55-60, 1980

26. Haskell W et al.: Cardiovascular responses to handgrip isometric exercise in patients following cardiac transplantation. Circulation Research (Supp I) 48: 156-161, 1981

27. Savin W et al.: Left ventricular response to isometric exercise in patients following cardiac transplantation. Circulation 61: 897-901, 1980

28. Kottke FJ, Stillwell GK, Lehmann JF: Krusen's Handbook of Physical Medicine and Rehabilitation, ed 3. Philadelphia, WB Saunders, 1982, pp 387, 969

29. Kinney MR, Pachia DR, Branigon, ME et al.: Care of the cardiac patient. In Fowkes VK, Andreoli KG, Zipes DP et al. (eds): Comprehensive Cardiac Care. St. Louis, CF Mosby, 1983, p 473

30. Borg GVA: Perceived Exertion: A note on history and methods. Med Sci Sports 5: 90-93, 1973

31. Fink A: Exercise Responses in the Transplant Population. APTA Cardiopulm Section Journal, Winter, 1986, pp 7-10

32. Borg GAV: Physical Performance and Perceived Exertion. Lund, Sweden, Gleerups, 1962

33. Prentice WE: Therapeutic Modalities In Sports Medicine. St. Louis, Times Mirror/Mosby College Publishing, 1986, p 122

Outpatient Rehabilitation
of the Cardiac Surgical Patient

Mary K. Laurenzi, PT

SUMMARY. Three different cardiac surgical patient populations are identified in this paper: the heart valve replacement (HVR) patient, the coronary artery bypass graft (CABG) patient, and the heart transplantation (HT) patient. Cardiac rehabilitation programs should provide comprehensive care to satisfy the patients' physical and psychosocial needs, and to offer education and support. The primary focus of this paper is outpatient rehabilitation, specifically exercise prescription and response in these patient populations. Such patients frequently share the same postoperative musculoskeletal problems resulting from the common sternotomy incision, requiring specialized exercises to regain strength, flexibility, and range of motion.

Cardiac surgical patients frequently are physically deconditioned prior to surgery as a result of their underlying cardiac disease. The patient with chronic valvular disease may be restricted by dyspnea on exertion resulting from underlying pulmonary edema. The patient with atherosclerotic coronary artery disease (CAD) may be limited by angina pectoris or a recent myocardial infarction. The patient with cardiomyopathy or end-stage coronary artery disease experiences chronic congestive heart failure and may complain about progressive shortness of breath, fatigue, or angina.

The patient's fitness level is decreased further by the effects of surgery. Several months are necessary for the body to recover physically and hemodynamically. Cardiopulmonary bypass and myocar-

---

Mary K. Laurenzi is affiliated with the Division of Physical and Occupational Therapy, Box 3965, Duke University Medical Center, Durham, NC.

dial preservation procedures traumatize the blood and can cause an increased bleeding tendency, denaturation of plasma protein, hemolysis, or obstruction to capillary blood flow.[1] While the long term effects of surgery usually allow the patient freedom to return to previous activities, the patient's immediate postoperative condition is one limited by fatigue, musculoskeletal pain, and decreased endurance. The ultimate goals of surgery and subsequent rehabilitation are to restore function and improve quality of life.[2-5]

Immediate postoperative inpatient rehabilitation is critical to prevent further deconditioning experienced with prolonged bedrest and inactivity. Equally important, but largely ignored, is outpatient rehabilitation following patient discharge from the hospital. This latter phase of rehabilitation is significant to the patient because it improves functional capacity and cardiovascular endurance, restores strength and flexibility, and promotes the self-confidence and self-esteem necessary to return to previous activities and occupational status.[6,7]

Depending on his medical history, physical status, and operative course, the patient may begin the program immediately following hospital discharge or shortly thereafter, preferably within one month postoperatively. Programs should include patient education to encourage lifestyle changes and risk factor modification, and education to inform patients about medications and their side effects.[6,8,9] Some programs offer support groups to assist patients in working out their psychosocial problems and in dealing with their heart disease and the subsequent surgery.

MEDICAL EVALUATION AND EXERCISE TESTING

Upon entering an outpatient program, each patient should have a thorough medical evaluation and a symptom-limited graded exercise test (SL-GXT). The medical evaluation should include a complete medical history, risk factor screening, cardiovascular examination, and laboratory blood tests. The SL-GXT may consist of a treadmill or a bicycle ergometer exercise test. The SL-GXT allows one to determine an individual's functional capacity and tolerance to exercise.[10,11] It also can be valuable in determining prognosis and indications for further diagnostic tests.[12] The patient's training heart rate range and metabolic equivalent of work (MET level) are calculated from the results of the SL-GXT.

EXERCISE PRESCRIPTION

The methods used to prescribe exercise parameters will vary from program to program. The following information outlines some general guidelines to consider when prescribing an exercise program for a cardiac surgical patient.

The mode of exercise training selected usually is one type of aerobic exercise (e.g., walking, jogging, biking, arm ergometry, swimming, or circuit weight training) or a combination of such exercises. To improve endurance, frequency of training should be at least three times per week,[13,14] although many programs exercise daily.[10,15,16] Intensity of exercise is usually 70 to 85% of the maximum heart rate reserve calculated from the SL-GXT.[6,7,13-15] In addition, the Borg rating of perceived exertion (RPE) scale also can be used to estimate intensity of training. An RPE of 13 ("somewhat hard") has been shown to correlate well with 70% of the maximum heart rate reserve.[16] Initially, duration of training may be brief (20 to 30 minutes); however, as the patient's endurance improves, he should exercise within his training heart rate range for 30 to 60 minutes.[10,16]

For proper warm-up and cool-down, a 5 to 15 minute period of calisthenics and stretching exercises should be incorporated into the training program. Warm-up exercises gradually increase circulation and body temperature, augmenting oxygen delivery to the working muscles. These exercises also improve joint flexibility, reduce the risk of musculoskeletal injury, and gradually increase coronary circulation. Cool-down exercises slowly lower the heart rate and blood pressure; they facilitate venous blood return to the heart, thus preventing cardiovascular complications resulting from blood pooling in the extremities. Cool-down exercises also help to prevent muscle cramping and soreness by facilitating removal of metabolic wastes.[17]

RESPONSE TO EXERCISE TRAINING

The HVR Patient

Although research is limited, beneficial effects of exercise training have been documented in the patient after HVR.[18,19] Serial oxygen consumption tests have shown an improvement in "cardiorespiratory fitness" in patients who engaged in physical training after HVR.[19] At a given workload, exercise training improves physical work capacity, decreases the rating of perceived exertion (RPE), and decreases the rate-pressure product (the heart rate times the systolic blood pressure) which indicates a decrease in myocardial oxygen consumption.[18]

The CABG Patient

The main purpose of myocardial revascularization is to restore blood flow to ischemic areas of the myocardium and thus relieve angina pectoris.[14] This makes it difficult to isolate the effects of exercise on myocardial perfusion after CABG surgery. Although long-term high-intensity exercise has enhanced myocardial perfusion in a few highly selected coronary artery disease patients, most individuals do not experience significant increase in coronary collateral circulation;[6,14] however, exercise training can increase maximum oxygen consumption by as much as 20%, and therefore significantly increase functional capacity.[6,14,20] Other benefits of exercise status-post CABG surgery include an increase in the cholesterol ratio of high density lipoprotein (HDL) to low density lipoprotein (LDL),[6,13] a reduction in triglycerides, and an improvement in glucose tolerance.[6,7] Exercise also lessens musculoskeletal discomfort, decreases anxiety and depression[7,13] and can lower percent body fat.[6,20] The physiological changes that occur with exercise training are well summarized by Wenger[6] as follows:

1. an increase in maximal cardiac output and oxygen consumption,
2. a lower resting heart rate and systolic blood pressure,
3. a lesser increase in heart rate and systolic blood pressure at any level of submaximal work,

4. a more rapid return to normal of the exercise heart rate,
5. decreased or absent angina pectoris at workloads that previously induced angina,
6. decreased or absent ECG ischemic (ST) changes at workloads that previously induced them.

The HT Patient

Response to exercise in the HT patient is quite different from that in the CABG patient or the HVR patient. When surgical orthotopic heart transplantation is performed, the majority of the patient's diseased heart is removed except for the posterior right and left atrial walls with the sinoatrial node and the venous connections. The donor heart is then anastomosed to the remaining atrial cuffs and to the vessels of the recipient's heart. In the surgical process of cardiac transplantation, the heart is denervated, losing its sympathetic stimulation via the autonomic nervous system. The cardiac muscle, however, continues to be affected by hormonal stimulation, specifically the release of catecholamines (epinephrine and norepinephrine) from the adrenal medullae. The strength and rate of cardiac muscle contraction is increased by the release of epinephrine, and the total arterial peripheral resistance is increased by the release of norepinephrine.[21]

With the absence of nervous innervation, the heart becomes supersensitive to the circulating catecholamines. This results in several physiological changes for the heart at rest and during exercise. First of all, the HT patient cannot experience angina because the heart is denervated.[21,22] Second, the HT patient has a higher than normal resting heart rate[23] due to lack of vagal stimulation.[21] Furthermore, the heart rate is unresponsive to autonomic manipulation such as the Valsalva maneuver or carotid massage.[21]

Exercise heart rate in the HT patient increases more slowly than normal as a result of the gradual release of circulating catecholamines.[21,23] Lack of sympathetic innervation results in maximum exercise heart rates that are less than normal peak values.[21,24] After exercise, a longer period is necessary for the heart rate to return to resting levels, because hormonal re-uptake is a slow process.[21] To avoid cardiovascular complications, the HT patient should do longer warm-up exercises, starting slowly and gradually increasing in intensity. Likewise, cool-down exercise also should be longer, decreasing in intensity until the heart rate approaches resting values.

Initially, the HT patient's stroke volume increases with exercise because more blood is being returned to the heart by exercising muscles (Starling's law);[21,22,25,26] later, it increases by the circulating catecholamines.[22,25,26] Cardiac output also increases with exercise but at less than normal peak values.[21,23,26,27] For most HT patients, ejection fraction increases with exercise, although it appears to be less than those of non-heart transplantation subjects.[21,28]

There are several differences between heart transplantation recipients and non-heart transplantation subjects. Oxygen consumption and physical work capacity are lower in the HT patient;[21,24] he reaches anaerobic threshold more quickly and has higher lactic acid accumulation post exercise.[21,24,25,29] He also shows a lower peak power output during exercise training.[24] Exercise duration is not significantly different from non-heart transplantation subjects.[23]

The HT recipient's ECG may show two separate P waves. One P wave may originate from the recipient's intact sinoatrial node but it cannot propagate across scar tissue. The other P wave, which comes from the donor's sinoatrial node, propagates to the atrioventricular node where a subsequent QRS complex follows.[21]

Kavanagh and associates showed that intense physical training of HT recipients in an outpatient setting resulted in increased lean body mass, increased maximal oxygen consumption, increased peak power, slightly lower resting heart rate, slightly higher maximal heart rate, and lower resting blood pressure. They did not find a significant change in exercise blood pressure.[24]

FLEXIBILITY – STRENGTHENING EXERCISES

Cardiac surgical patients require exercises in addition to the endurance exercises of walking, jogging, and biking. During surgery, a sternotomy is performed and the chest wall is separated to open the mediastinal area. This procedure results in many soft tissue structures being injured, for example muscles, tendons, and ligaments. Furthermore, when the internal mammary arteries are used for CABG, the patient's chest wall is stretched apart even further. The sternum is wired back together in approximately three areas and bone healing occurs over a six to eight week period.

During the postoperative rehabilitation phase, each patient should be evaluated for sternal instability, often recognized as a sternal "click." A sternal "click" may be detected by palpation with an open hand placed gently over the sternum. If the sternum is unstable, it will "click," "pop," or "grate" when the patient does asymmetrical movements. The patient with a sternal "click" can continue to exercise provided that the exercises do not cause sternal movement. Therefore, the exercises should be symmetrical (i.e., bilateral shoulder flexion) and twisting type exercises should be avoided. The patient may not be able to do upper extremity exercises on arm ergometers or the Airdyne ergometer until the "click" has resolved. Most sternal "clicks" resolve by four to eight weeks postoperatively.

After surgery, the superficial incision often becomes sensitive to touch secondary to injured nerve endings. Combined with strained muscles, this often leads to poor postural habits of a protracted shoulder girdle and a forward head. It is important, therefore, that the cardiac surgical patient receives an exercise program that restores strength, flexibility, range of motion, and normal posture. Stretching and strengthening exercises should concentrate on the muscles of the upper extremities, shoulder girdle and thorax. To promote normal posture, stretching of the pectoralis muscles is important. A comprehensive exercise program should include exercises for the back, abdomen, and lower extremities as well. Free weights, Theraband, and weightlifting equipment such as Universal or Nautilus machines can be used.

Weight training can be performed safely by cardiac patients,[30,31] including cardiac surgical patients,[32-35] and can be accomplished without the patient experiencing significant ST segment depression, angina, or significant ventricular arrhythmias.[30,32,34,35] However, research is lacking regarding the hemodynamic response to weight training in the heart transplantation patient. Depending on the patient's medical status, age and fitness level, weight training can be done as a low level program with low weights and high repetition, or it can be done more intensely such as circuit weight training.

Circuit weight training implies that an individual develops both strength and cardiovascular endurance by training at 60 to 80% of his maximum heart rate.[30-32,36] It involves a workout time of at least 20 to 30 minutes daily to three times per week, during which the individual completes two to three circuits of resistive exercises on 10 to 15 special weight machines. The individual does 12 to 15 repetitions on each machine at 40 to 50% maximum lift, taking minimal rest periods of 15 to 30 seconds between machines.[31,36] Results show an increase in strength, an increase in lean body mass, improved endurance,[30-32,36] as well as an increase in self-perceived ability to accomplish similar lifting tasks.[33]

CONCLUSION

The cardiac surgical patient requires outpatient rehabilitation following hospitalization for several reasons: to regain endurance, strength, flexibility and range of motion, to restore normal posture, and to reestablish self-confidence and self-esteem. Inpatient rehabilitation does not allow adequate time to accomplish such goals. Response to exercise varies from the HVR patient and the CABG patient to the HT patient. Nevertheless, all three patient populations benefit from continued exercise training and they report an improved quality of life as well as increased functional capacity when following such programs.

REFERENCES

1. Gibbon JH, Sabiston DC, Spencer FC: Surgery of the Chest, ed 3. Philadelphia, WB Saunders Company, 1976

2. Stanton BA, Jenkins CD, Savageau JA et al.: Functional benefits following coronary artery bypass graft surgery. Ann. Thorac. Surg. 37:286-290, 1984

3. Christopherson LK, Griepp RB, Stinson EB: Rehabilitation after cardiac transplantation. JAMA 236:2082-2084, 1976

4. Christopherson LK: Cardiac transplantation: A psychological perspective. Circulation 75:57-62, 1987

5. Pere E, Saraste M, Inberg M et al.: Clinical findings and return to work after heart valve replacement. Scand. J. Rehab. Med. 16:65-70, 1984

6. Wenger NK: Rehabilitation of the coronary patient: Status 1986. Prog. Cardiovasc. Dis. 29:181-199, 1986

7. Oberman A, Kouchoukos NT: Role of exercise after coronary artery bypass surgery. Cardiovasc. Clinics 9:155-172, 1978

8. Grady KL, Bucjley DJ, Cisar NS et al.: Patient perception of cardiovascular surgical patient education. Heart Lung 17:349-355, 1988

9. Marshall J, Penckofer S, Llewellyn J: Structured postoperative teaching and knowledge and compliance of patients who had coronary artery bypass surgery. Heart Lung 15:76-82, 1986

10. Pollock ML, Wilmore JH, Fox SM: Exercise in Health and Disease: Evaluation and Prescription for Prevention and Rehabilitation. Philadelphia, WB Saunders Company, 1984

11. Hamm LF, Stull GA, Wolfe DR: Graded exercise testing early after myocardial revascularization surgery. Arch. Phys. Med. Rehabil. 68:165-169, 1987

12. American College of Sports Medicine: Guidelines for Graded Exercise Testing, ed 3. Philadelphia, Lea and Febiger, 1986

13. Murray CG, Beller GA: Cardiac rehabilitation following coronary artery bypass surgery. Am. Heart J. 105:1009-1018, 1983

14. Oldridge NB, Nagle FJ, Balke B et al.: Aortocoronary bypass surgery: Effects of surgery and 32 months of physical conditioning on treadmill performance. Arch. Phys. Med. Rehabil. 59:268-275, 1978

15. Metier CP, Pollock ML, Graves JE: Exercise prescription for coronary artery bypass graft surgery patient. J. Cardiopulmonary Rehabil. 6:85-103, 1986

16. Pollock ML: Exercise regimes after myocardial revascularization surgery: Rationale and results, in Wenger NK, Brest AN, (eds): Exercise and the Heart, ed 2. Philadelphia, FA Davis, 1984

17. Cornett SJ, Watson JR: Cardiac Rehabilitation: An Interdisciplinary Team Approach. New York, Wiley Medical, 1984

18. Sire S: Physical training and occupational rehabilitation after aortic valve replacement. Eur. Heart J. 8:1215-1220, 1987

19. Newell, JP, Kappagoda CT, Stoker JB et al.: Physical training after heart valve replacement. Br. Heart J. 44:638-649, 1980

20. LaFontaine T, Bruckerhoff D: The efficacy and risk of intense aerobic circuit training in coronary artery disease patients following bypass surgery. Phys. Sportsmed 15:141-149, 1987

21. Fick AW: Exercise response in the transplant population. Cardiopulmonary Record 1:7-10, 1986

22. Arthur EK: Rehabilitation of potential and cardiac transplant recipients. Cardiopulmonary Record 1:11-13, 1986

23. Pflugfelder PW, Purves PD, McKenzie FN et al.: Cardiac dynamics during supine exercise in cyclosporine-treated orthotopic heart transplant recipients: Assessment by radionuclide angiography. J. Am. Coll. Cardio. 10:336-341, 1987

24. Kavanagh T, Yacoub MH, Mertens DJ et al.: Cardiorespiratory responses to exercise training after orthotopic cardiac transplantation. Circulation 77:162-171, 1988

25. Degre SG, Niset GL, DeSmet JM et al.: Cardiorespiratory response to

early exercise testing after orthotopic cardiac transplantation. Am. J. Cardio. 60:926-928, 1987

26. Pope SE, Stinson EB, Daughters GT et al.: Exercise response of the denervated heart in long-term cardiac transplant recipients. Am. J. Cardiol. 46:213-218, 1980

27. Pflugfelder PW, McKenzie FN, Kostuk WJ: Hemodynamic profiles at rest and during supine exercise after orthotopic cardiac transplantation. Am. J. Cardio. 61:1328-1333, 1988

28. Verani MS, George SE, Leon CA et al.: Systolic and diastolic ventricular performance at rest and during exercise in heart transplant recipients. J. Heart Transplant 7:145-151, 1988

29. Niset G, Poortmans JR, Leclercq R et al.: Metabolic implications during a 20-km run after heart transplantation. Int. J. Sports Med. 6:340-343, 1985

30. Butler RM, Beirwaltes WH, Rogers FJ: The cardiovascular response to circuit weight training in patients with cardiac disease. J. Cardiopulmonary Rehabil. 7:402-409, 1987

31. Keleman MH, Stewart KJ: Circuit weight training: A new direction for cardiac rehabilitation. Sports Med. 2:385-388, 1985

32. Keleman MH, Stewart KJ, Gillilan RE et al.: Circuit weight training in cardiac patients. J. Am. Coll. Cardiol. 7:38-42, 1986

33. Ewart CK, Stewart KJ, Gillilan RE et al.: Self-efficacy mediates strength gains during circuit weight training in men with coronary artery disease. Med. Sci. Sports 18:531-540, 1986

34. Haslam DR, McCartney N, McKelvie RS et al.: Direct measurement of arterial blood pressure during formal weightlifting in cardiac patients. J. Cardiopulmonary Rehabil. 8:213-225, 1988

35. Vander LB, Franklin BA, Wrisley D et al.: Acute cardiovascular responses to Nautilus exercise in cardiac patients: Implications for exercise training. Ann. Sports Med. 2:165-169, 1986

36. Gettman LR, Pollock ML: Circuit weight training: A critical review of its physiological benefits. Phys. Sports Med. 9:44-60, 1981